Powerful Habits for Aging Well

Quarto.com
© 2025 Quarto Publishing Group USA Inc.
Text © 2025 Editors of Fair Winds Press

First Published in 2025 by Fair Winds Press, an imprint of The Quarto Group, 100 Cummings Center, Suite 265-D, Beverly, MA 01915, USA.
T (978) 282-9590 F (978) 283-2742

All rights reserved. No part of this book may be reproduced in any form without written permission of the copyright owners. All images in this book have been reproduced with the knowledge and prior consent of the artists concerned, and no responsibility is accepted by producer, publisher, or printer for any infringement of copyright or otherwise, arising from the contents of this publication. Every effort has been made to ensure that credits accurately comply with the information supplied. We apologize for any inaccuracies that may have occurred and will resolve inaccurate or missing information in a subsequent reprinting of the book.

Fair Winds Press titles are also available at discount for retail, wholesale, promotional, and bulk purchase. For details, contact the Special Sales Manager by email at specialsales@quarto.com or by mail at The Quarto Group, Attn: Special Sales Manager, 100 Cummings Center, Suite 265-D, Beverly, MA 01915, USA.

29 28 27 26 25   1 2 3 4 5

ISBN: 978-0-7603-9722-0

Digital edition published in 2025
eISBN: 978-0-7603-9723-7

Library of Congress Cataloging-in-Publication Data available

Design and illustration: Timothy Samara

Printed in China

The information in this book is for educational purposes only. It is not intended to replace the advice of a physician or medical practitioner. Please see your health-care provider before beginning any new health program.

Powerful Habits for Aging Well

Strategies for Longevity and Health

FAIR WINDS

Contents

INTRODUCTIONS

The Powerful Habits Series • *8*

Introduction to This Book • *9*

01 Powerful Habits to Turn Back the Clock on Your Face • *10*

Habit #1: Prevent and Erase Age-Related Wrinkles and More • *12*

Habit #2: Omega-3 Fatty Acids and Antioxidants = Younger-Looking Skin • *16*

Habit #3: Destress to Look Younger • *19*

Habit #4: Use Treatments at Home to Take Years Off Your Face, Teeth, and Hair • *22*

02 Powerful Habits to Turn Back the Clock on Your Body • *28*

Habit #1: Feast on Metabolism-Boosting Foods • *30*

Habit #2: Escape the Stress-Fat Cycle for a More Youthful Waistline • *32*

Habit #3: Lose Weight While You Sleep • *34*

Habit #4: Rev Up Midlife Metabolism, Build Strength, and Improve Flexibility and Balance • *36*

03 Powerful Habits to Turn Back the Clock on Your Brain · *42*

Habit #1: Eat a Diet to Cool Inflammation and Keep Your Brain Young · *44*

Habit #2: Manage Depression and Stress to Minimize Brain Aging · *47*

Habit #3: Sharpen Mental Focus with Mind-Body Techniques · *52*

Habit #4: Challenge Your Brain to Improve Cognition as You Get Older · *54*

Habit #5: Tap Antioxidant Supplements and More to Boost Brain Health · *56*

04 Powerful Habits to Turn Back the Clock on Your Bones and Joints · *58*

Habit #1: Achieve and Keep a Healthy Weight to Reduce Joint Stress and Protect Your Bones · *60*

Habit #2: Boost Bone Building Beyond Calcium and Vitamin D · *63*

Habit #3: Diet Don'ts for Healthy Bones and Joints for Life · *68*

Habit #4: Use Natural Remedies to Strengthen Joints · *70*

Habit #5: Reduce Midlife Joint Pain with Alternative Therapies · *73*

05 Powerful Habits to Turn Back the Clock on Your Heart · *76*

Habit #1: Lower Your Cholesterol and Blood Pressure Naturally · *78*

Habit #2: Get the Nutrients You Need to Stave Off Heart Disease · *81*

Habit #3: Tame Your Emotions (Anger, Depression, and Stress) to Take Years Off Your Ticker · *84*

Habit #4: Keep Your Heart Young and Strong with These Supplements · *87*

06 Powerful Habits to Turn Back the Clock on Your Immune System · *90*

Habit #1: Use Mind-Body Therapies to Stop Aging Stress · *92*

Habit #2: Don't Skimp on Sleep as You Get Older · *95*

Habit #3: See the Glass as Half-Full to Bolster Immunity · *98*

Habit #4: Supercharge Your Diet with Immune-Boosting Foods · *102*

Habit #5: Supercharge Your Immunity with Nutrients and Herbs · *105*

07 Powerful Habits to Turn Back the Clock on Your Sex Life · *108*

Habit #1: Address Underlying Health Issues for a Longer Love Life · *110*

Habit #2: Maintain Sexual Confidence as You Age · *112*

Habit #3: Practice Mindfulness to Renew Romance · *115*

Habit #4: Exercise to Reverse Age-Related Sexual Problems · *118*

Habit #5: Dial Back Stress to Rev Up Your Love Life · *120*

Habit #6: Be Honest about Shifting Needs and Desires · *122*

Habit #7: Take Herbs and Supplements to Restore a Sexual Spark · *126*

08 Powerful Habits to Turn Back the Clock for More Energy · *128*

Habit #1: Don't Let Stress Slow You Down · *130*

Habit #2: Use Newton's Law: Keep Moving to Counteract Fatigue · *132*

Habit #3: Eat to Sustain All-Day Energy · *134*

Habit #4: Perk Up with Safe Supplements and Practices to Feel Younger · *136*

Habit #5: Reenergize by Finding Renewed Purpose · *139*

09 Powerful Habits: Important Dos and Don'ts to Slow the Aging Process · *142*

Habit #1: Don't Smoke or Vape to Live Longer and Better · *144*

Habit #2: Conquer Couch Potato Syndrome to Stay Fit for Life · *147*

Habit #3: Don't Let Your BMI Creep Too High in Midlife · *148*

Habit #4: Steer Clear of Chronic Stress to Prevent Premature Aging · *151*

Habit #5: Don't Let Your Genes Shorten Your Life · *153*

Habit #6: Build and Maintain a Strong Social Network to Live Longer · *155*

Index · *158*

THE POWERFUL HABITS SERIES

habit /hăb·ĭt/ noun

1. A recurrent, often unconscious pattern of behavior that is acquired through frequent repetition.

2. An established disposition of the mind or character.

3. Customary manner or practice.

The American Heritage® Dictionary of the English Language, 5th Edition

What Can You Achieve in Five Minutes?

What can you achieve in five minutes? Plenty. **Powerful Habits** is a new series that focuses on practical, immediately applicable strategies that can uplevel your health and life starting today. Instead of wading through hundreds of pages, numerous steps, and a complicated program, Powerful Habits gives you quick-take advice, much of which can be done in five minutes or less.

What we do, we often become. Much of our behavior is unconscious and bad habits have a way of taking root without us noticing it. But you can counteract this by making good habits a part of your day and your life. It's like putting money in the bank. If you do it consistently, you'll build wealth through your actions and the interest that accumulates.

It's the same way when you adopt habits each day to help you look and feel younger. Even better, practicing habits consistently produces even more benefits over time. For example, say you add kiwi fruits to your diet. You'll feel better right away because you know you're adding antioxidants from vitamin C to fight free radicals and the aging they can cause. Over time, eating foods like this will also have protective effects against many of the chronic diseases associated with aging. So, you're younger today and tomorrow. It's a win-win! Inside this book, you'll find new habits that you can read and put into practice in just a few minutes each day. You'll find that it's super easy to dip in and out of this book to easily select habits and see results in real-time. Open the book, read a spread, and apply the advice to your life. Your better self is five minutes away!

Introduction to This Book

Who doesn't want to live a longer, healthier, and happier life? My hope is that with this book, you can use these safe, effective, and scientifically proven tips to slow the aging process in a real and lasting way. The good news is that you don't have to overhaul your entire life—even making one or two changes can help you look and feel younger in just a few days or weeks. After you get a few tips under your belt, add a few more to build on your success. It really is that easy, and whether you're thirty, sixty, or ninety, it's never too late (or too early!) to start.

Of course, on some days the healthier choices are easier to make than on others. But often, if you do one good thing for yourself, you're much more motivated to keep it up. Think of each day as filled with opportunities to take care of yourself and ensure your good health for the long haul. The beauty of this book is that you have so many antiaging options to choose from; if you don't feel like exercising one day, you can meet a friend for lunch instead and know that you're still keeping yourself young.

You might be surprised at all the ways you can slow the aging process. There are so many ways to turn back the clock. To be sure, your quickest path to antiaging is adopting healthy habits such as eating more fruits and vegetables and exercising. But volunteering, cultivating an optimistic outlook, and practicing forgiveness also play a big part. And did you know lifestyle changes like cutting back on refined carbs are twice as effective at preventing diabetes as medications?

Available to everyone, lifestyle changes such as these carry virtually no risk of side effects, and in many cases they're actually more effective than drugs, surgery, or other medical interventions. They are also, by far, the least expensive ways to maintain or restore good health. That translates into less time in the doctor's office, fewer medications, lower medical bills, and the good health and energy to keep doing the things you love for decades to come. So start reading and begin turning back the clock today.

Powerful Habits to Turn Back the Clock on Your Face

01

As we age the signs (unfortunately) show up on our face. There's really no place to hide. But if you make skin care practices for younger skin a priority, you can protect, revitalize, and even reverse the signs of aging.

What's your Skin Care IQ? >

Which of the following do you want to do?

Protect your skin from sun damage that makes your skin age faster.

Reverse Sahara-like dry skin that makes you look older.

Stop fretting about wrinkles and begin to erase them.

Learn how you can prevent wrinkles.

Choose foods that will keep your skin looking younger.

Minimize the effects that stress can have on your skin.

Find less expensive ways to have younger-looking skin, teeth, and hair.

* If you answered [YES] to any of these questions, read on for habits that can prevent and erase the inevitable signs of aging and turn back the clock on your face.

HABIT #1
Prevent and Erase Age-Related Wrinkles and More

Protect your skin from sun damage that makes your skin age faster.

YES

UVA and UVB rays create free radicals that damage healthy skin cells, break down elastin and speed up collagen loss, and lead to wrinkles. This is why sunscreens are commonly recommended.

But in 2021, the FDA (Food and Drug Administration) reviewed sixteen ingredients commonly found in sunscreen and found only two as being safe and effective: zinc oxide and titanium dioxide. However, zinc oxide can become toxic after two hours on the skin, and although it's a low risk for most, titanium dioxide may cause cancer when inhaled. The other common ingredients, including oxybenzone and avobenzone, can be hormone disruptors and can cause skin irritation. Given all of this and the fact that you're supposed to apply sunscreen daily, it's smart to look for alternatives.

A 2018 study in the medical journal *Nutrients* showed that taking 4 milligrams of astaxanthin (the red carotenoid that makes shrimp and salmon pink) can help prevent ultraviolet (UV)-induced sunburn. Astaxanthin has antioxidant properties that counterbalance the oxidation caused by exposure to UV rays that results in inflammation. If you have a chronic medical condition, check with your health practitioner before taking it.

Eating foods high in astaxanthin such as shrimp, crab, and wild-caught salmon may also offer benefits. Omega-3 fatty acid choices like fatty cold-water fish and antioxidant-rich brightly colored fruits and vegetables can lower inflammation caused by sunburn. Be sure and take astaxanthin in conjunction with a sunscreen that's at least an SPF 30 and mineral based. The Environmental Working Group has a list of best sunscreens on their website: **www.ewg.org/sunscreen.**

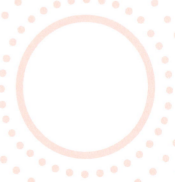

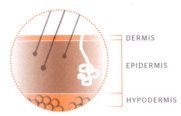

Reverse Sahara-like dry skin that makes you look older.

 YES

As you get older, your skin undergoes changes at every level. The top layer (the epidermis) thins and loses protective fatty substances called *lipids,* making skin drier and less able to fight off infection. Arid climates or the dry air in winter can aggravate parched skin even more.

Dry skin can feel tight and uncomfortable, accentuate wrinkles, and look flaky and ashy. Also, as you age, the inner layer (the dermis)—made of the collagen and elastic tissues that keep your skin firm and plump—begins to break down, leading to wrinkles. These changes mean your skin doesn't bounce back from injury as quickly. These habits can help repair and rejuvenate your skin:

Hydrate Your Skin with Hyaluronic Acid (aka sodium hyaluronate)

Hyaluronic acid, which is found naturally in the skin, calms itchiness and irritation, plumps and smooths skin, and restores a youthful, dewy look. A 2004 study in *Skin Pharmacology and Physiology* noted that hyaluronic acid boosts production of cells that make and secrete collagen, at the same time shoring up skin's structure.

Hyaluronic acid moisturizes skin from the inside, increases elasticity, calms inflammation, and scavenges skin-damaging free radicals. As you get older, you produce less hyaluronic acid, which can lead to dry skin and wrinkles.

The good news? Applying it topically seems to restore some of those benefits, plumping and firming skin almost immediately. You can find topical hyaluronic acid in moisturizers at all price points in serums, creams, gels, and so on, often alongside other antiaging ingredients to give you multiple benefits in one bottle. If you have sensitive skin, choose a moisturizer that is fragrance free. If you're acne prone, use an oil-free moisturizer that's noncomedogenic and nonacnegenic to banish breakouts.

Apply a moisturizer with hyaluronic acid after you wash your face with a mild, soap-free cleanser to lock in moisture. Dry skin? Wash your face at night and just wet your skin and dry it in the morning.

Stop fretting about wrinkles and begin to erase them.

✳ YES

Use Retin-A to Protect against Collagen Breakdown and Repair Collagen

While hyaluronic acid moisturizes the skin, Retin-A repairs it. In a 2009 study, French researchers found that with nine months of regular application, a 0.1 percent retinol treatment improved under-eye wrinkles, fine lines, and skin tone. Retin-A protects against collagen breakdown and repairs collagen and elastic fibers, restoring collagen production by about 80 percent over ten to twelve months of daily use. It also improves wrinkles and skin texture and color. Over-the-counter products with retinols offer more subtle benefits. For a more noticeable difference, see your dermatologist for prescription strength Retin-A.

Retin-A can irritate the skin, so start with a small amount every other day and build up to daily application. It increases your sensitivity to sunlight, so wear sunscreen when you use it. Retin-A cream at 0.05 percent helps heal mild to moderate photodamage as well.

Apply Peptides and Other Topical Treatments at Bedtime

In 2017, German researchers reviewed the many antiaging benefits of applying topical peptides in the medical journal *Cosmetics*. That's because when collagen breaks down, it forms short chains of amino acids called *peptides* that spur skin to repair itself. Applying peptides topically at night may trick your skin into thinking it needs to make more collagen. Peptides typically bind water and, therefore, help hydrate skin. That especially benefits aging skin, since skin gets drier as you mature and dry skin accentuates wrinkles. Other effective topical treatments include formulations with antioxidant vitamins, such as C, E, and A; green tea; coenzyme Q10 and alpha hydroxy acids (AHAs), which boost collagen, and hydrate and exfoliate skin.

**MAKE IT A HABIT:
TIPS TO FIGHT WRINKLES**

Take 4-milligram capsules of astaxanthin and use a mineral-based sunscreen to prevent UV damage to your skin. Incorporate hyaluronic acid, Retin-A, and other topicals that can help make skin look younger into your daily skin care routine. Adopt wrinkle prevention habits to prevent aging.

Learn how you can prevent wrinkles.

YES

Wear sunglasses. Sunglasses with 100 percent UV protection shield eyes and the surrounding delicate skin from sun damage. Wear them outdoors, even in winter. In fact, sunlight reflecting off snow can be even brighter than the summer sun.

Avoid repetitive movements. Squinting can lead to crow's feet, and furrowing your brow, pursing your lips, or frowning which can lead to wrinkles. Repetitive facial movements form grooves beneath the skin's surface every time the facial muscles contract. That repeated wear and tear causes changes in the connective tissue and breaks down the extracellular matrix, skin's support structure. As you age, your skin can't snap back into place as easily, and over time those grooves become wrinkles, according to the American Academy of Dermatology. If you need glasses, get them and wear them. You won't need to squint to read the fine print.

Plug in a humidifier to moisturize mature skin. When we age, the outermost layer of your epidermis (the stratum corneum) loses lipids, the fatty substances that protect and keep your skin moist. Dry skin can make wrinkles more noticeable and lead to flaky, ashy skin—quite the opposite of the dewy complexion of your youth.

A 2007 study in the *Journal of Biomedical Optics* found that increasing the relative humidity of the air causes skin to plump up, potentially diminishing wrinkles. To combat dry air, use a humidifier in your bedroom at night or place a tray of water on top of a radiator. The heat will cause the water to evaporate and add moisture back into the air. Keeping well-watered houseplants nearby will also raise humidity. An inexpensive hygrometer, available at hardware stores or online, can track humidity levels; aim for 50 percent humidity, and no less than 30 percent, the amount at which skin starts to feel uncomfortably dry.

Sleep the right way. The American Academy of Dermatology notes that people who sleep on their sides or stomach tend to smoosh their faces into their pillows. If you sleep in the same position every night, sleep lines can form along the chin and cheeks (if you're a side sleeper) or the forehead (if you sleep facedown). As your skin loses elasticity with age, the lines stick around even when you're not resting your head on a pillow. The answer? Sleep on your back if you can, or at least vary your sleeping position from day to day.

HABIT #2
Omega-3 Fatty Acids and Antioxidants = Younger-Looking Skin

Choose foods that will keep your skin looking younger.
YES

Skin is the body's largest living organ, and it needs top-notch nourishment to function and look its best. While a healthy diet filled with fruits and vegetables, whole grains, lean protein, and good fats will work wonders for your appearance, a few skin superstars are worth working into your diet for their antiaging benefits.

Omega-3 and Omega-6 Fatty Acids Protect against Skin Aging

Sure, omega-3s are beneficial for heart health and the brain, but they're also critical for skin health and can fight signs of aging, along with omega-6s. These essential fatty acids calm inflammation and irritation caused by free radicals. They keep cell membranes fluid and flexible and normalize oil production by creating protective lipids (fatty substances) in your skin's topmost layer—especially helpful as your skin gets drier with age, and since dry skin makes wrinkles more noticeable. Omega-3s and omega-6s also defend against cell damage and assist in repair, keeping skin resilient. A 2006 review of studies concluded that consuming omega-3s can actually protect skin from sun damage as well.

Omega-3s and omega-6s are called *essential fatty acids* because our bodies can't make them, so we have to get them through diet. Omega-6s are abundant in foods like eggs, vegetable oils, poultry, and grains, and most people consume more than enough. The trick is getting enough omega-3s.

Omega-3s are a group of several nutrients, including eicosapentaenoic acid (EPA) and docosahexaenoic acid (DHA). Fatty, cold-water fish like wild salmon, lake trout, albacore tuna, herring, anchovies, and sardines are among the best sources. Surprisingly, grass-fed beef also offers a respectable amount. Omega-3–fortified eggs and other fortified foods are another option. Walnuts, ground flaxseed, and soy foods like tofu provide another omega-3 known as alpha-linolenic acid (ALA), which the body can use to make EPA and DHA. Broccoli, cabbage, and other leafy greens also supply small amounts of ALA.

Add Age-Fighting Antioxidants

Like omega-3s and omega-6s, antioxidant vitamins A, C, and E fight free radicals that can damage skin and lead to wrinkles, or even skin cancer. Topical antioxidants get a lot of press, but your primary goal should be to get enough through diet. Brightly colored fruits and vegetables, such as avocados, broccoli, carrots, kiwis, nuts and seeds, oranges, red and green peppers, spinach, and strawberries are super sources.

It can be tough to get enough vitamin E from foods, but you should talk to your doctor if you're thinking about supplementing, since vitamin E can act as a blood thinner, and high levels may interfere with cholesterol-lowering drugs. If you choose to supplement with vitamin E, take 400 IU of mixed natural tocopherols daily. D-alpha tocopherol is the natural form; avoid synthetic dl-alpha tocopherol.

> **MAKE IT A HABIT:**
> **EAT FATTY ACIDS AND ANTIOXIDANTS**
>
> Eat two 3- to 4-ounce servings of oily fish a week.
>
> If your diet falls short, talk to your doctor about taking a fish oil supplement that contains 500 milligrams or more of EPA and DHA or one made from algae that has 400 to 600 milligrams of DHA.
>
> Make it a habit to add antioxidant- and mineral-rich foods to breakfast, lunch, dinner, and snacks.

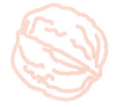
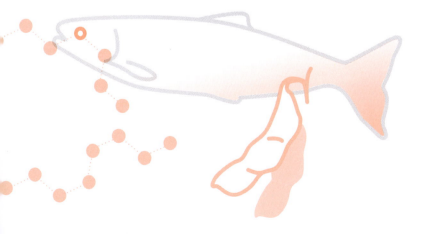

Include Minerals in Your Antiaging Diet

A 2009 study noted that people with high levels of selenium in their blood reduced their risk of skin cancer by about 60 percent. Its antioxidant action helps prevent premature skin aging, and it encourages vitamin E absorption as well. Good sources include brown rice, seafood, garlic, eggs, and Brazil nuts.

Another multitasker, zinc, protects your skin from sun damage and works with vitamin C to make collagen. A zinc deficiency can trigger breakouts, lead to hair loss, and cause rough skin or rashes. Food sources include oysters, legumes (such as beans and peas), red meat, pecans, and pumpkin seeds. If you don't eat many animal foods, you might want to supplement, but the National Institutes of Health (NIH) Office of Dietary Supplements recommends getting no more than 40 milligrams per day.

Skin Renewal Shopping List

Use this list to make it easier to add omega-3s, omega-6s, antioxidants, and nutrients to your meals and snacks.

Omega-3s:

Fatty, cold-water fish like wild salmon, lake trout, albacore tuna, herring, anchovies, and sardines; grass-fed beef; omega-3-fortified eggs; other fortified foods; walnuts, ground flaxseed; soy foods like tofu; and broccoli, cabbage, and other leafy greens

Omega-6s:

Eggs, vegetable oils, poultry, and grains

Antioxidants:

Brightly colored fruits and vegetables, such as avocados, broccoli, carrots, kiwis, nuts and seeds, oranges, red and green peppers, spinach, and strawberries

Selenium:

Brown rice, seafood, garlic, eggs, and Brazil nuts

Zinc:

Oysters, legumes (such as beans and peas), red meat, pecans, and pumpkin seeds

HABIT #3
Destress to Look Younger

Minimize the effects that stress can have on your skin.

YES

Your eyes may be the window to your soul, but your skin is a pretty good indicator of your emotional health. In fact, experts are realizing that the connection between emotions and skin is so strong that they've coined a term for this growing field: *psychodermatology*.

Dermatologists have long recognized that stress can make your skin more sensitive and worsen conditions such as acne, eczema, and rosacea, but research reveals that it can also add years to your appearance. For example, stress dehydrates skin, and a 2009 study in the *Journal of Biomechanics* found that reducing moisture in the skin's top layer by 11 percent produces wrinkles that are 25 to 85 percent larger. Stress also breaks down skin-firming collagen and slows your body's ability to make more collagen. Additionally, stress can increase skin inflammation, leading to itchiness, flushing, and uneven skin tone.

If that weren't bad enough, in addition to the direct effects of stress on your skin, anxiety often causes people to neglect good skin care habits or abuse their skin by rubbing, pulling, or picking at it. But before you resort to hiding your head under a paper bag, there are plenty of ways you can tame tension and stop its aging effects on your skin. Feeling good about your skin's appearance may reduce stress and anxiety in other parts of your life as well. Here are some stress-busting, skin-saving tips.

THE BENEFITS OF YOGA NIDRA

Yoga Nidra, or "yogic sleep," is the perfect antidote if you're stressed out. This practice activates the relaxation response through your parasympathetic nervous system. You can also do this by slow, deep breathing, progressive relaxation, and meditation. It's the easiest yoga ever because you do it lying down. Yoga Nidra involves a body scan, or what's known as a rotation of consciousness. As you tune in as each body part is noted, you let go, and soon you'll feel relaxed from head to toe. Find Yoga Nidra meditations that take a few minutes or an hour-plus if you have more time.

JOURNAL PAGE

Writing about your frustrations, irritations, and stressors each day can help you put them into perspective. Set a timer for five minutes and get it out on the page. You'll feel better.

Su

Mo

Tu

We

Th

Fr

Sa

MAKE IT A HABIT: REDUCE STRESS

Feeling stressed? Set a reminder on your calendar or your phone to remind you to do face yoga, yoga Nidra, 4-7-8 breathing, or breathing exercises throughout the day.

Practice Face Yoga

Face yoga relieves tension and may also help you look younger by strengthening and toning facial muscles through a series of exercises and stretches. In a small study at Northwestern University published in *JAMA Dermatology* in 2018, participants aged forty to sixty-five were first instructed in thirty-two facial exercises and then performed them daily for thirty minutes for weeks one to eight, and three to four times a week for weeks nine to twenty. The outcome was improved upper and lower cheek fullness. You can find facial yoga courses online or take in-person instruction from a certified face yoga teacher.

STUDY SHOWS EXERCISE LOWERS STRESS AND IMPROVES MOOD

A 2007 study in *Biological Research for Nursing* looked at adults over age sixty and noted that thirty minutes of walking at 60 percent of their maximum heart rate (considered moderate exercise) significantly lowered stress and improved mood after ten weeks. In addition, a 2009 study in the *European Journal of Applied Physiology* measured circulation to the skin in post-menopausal women after they had exercised for twenty-four, thirty-six, and forty-eight weeks, and found that circulation continued to improve the longer the women had been exercising.

Use 4-7-8 Breathing to Revive Aging Skin

Breathing practices not only help you relax but also help you inhale more oxygen, which refreshes and rejuvenates your skin. Extra oxygen also tells your skin to ramp up production of collagen, which plumps your skin and makes wrinkles less noticeable. This simple breathing technique from Dr. Andrew Weil, M.D., an expert in natural healing and healthy aging, does the trick whenever you're stressed and need to relax. He suggests first placing the tip of your tongue just behind your upper front teeth. Keep it there throughout the exercise. Exhale completely through your mouth, making a whooshing sound. Inhale quietly through your nose while you count to four. Hold your breath for seven counts, then exhale through your mouth (making the whoosh sound again) for a count of eight. Repeat the cycle four times. Kiss those worry lines goodbye!

Exercise to Erase Stress and Keep Skin Young

Exercise is perhaps the best stress reliever there is, and it offers both short- and long-term benefits. Even as little as ten minutes of movement can stop stress in its tracks, which is a pretty remarkable return on investment.

For immediate impact, exercise helps burn off extra energy when tension has you tied in knots, and it boosts circulation to bring nutrients to the skin, remove toxins, and improve skin tone. In the long run, it helps keep your stress hormones balanced, allowing you to stay calm even in the face of chronic chaos.

In 2008, University of Colorado researchers performed a series of animal studies showing that regular exercise modifies the way the body responds to the stress hormone cortisol, ultimately reducing the amount the body and brain are exposed to. Reducing your exposure to cortisol could translate to keeping skin better hydrated, boosting collagen production, and calming inflammation.

To get the best stress-busting effects of exercise, you should enjoy it, so how you get moving—a brisk walk or run, lifting weights, yoga or stretching, dancing, or hitting a punching bag—is up to you.

HABIT #4
Use Treatments at Home to Take Years Off Your Face, Teeth, and Hair

Find less expensive ways to have younger-looking skin, teeth, and hair.

YES

The American Academy of Dermatology notes that at-home treatments "can be safe when they have been thoroughly tested for this type of self-use"—as long as you follow the package directions. Here's what you need to know if you'd like to try them on your own.

Expose Your Skin to Red Light Treatments

Research published in the medical journal *Photomedicine Laser Surgery* in 2018 shows that red light therapy (RLT) or photobiomodulation improves collagen density, reduces fine lines and wrinkles, and softens rough skin. It also may reduce inflammation and improve skin elasticity. You can tap into the power of this therapy by wearing an RLT mask, lying in an RLT therapy bed, sitting in front of a red light panel, or using an RLT wand. Look for an FDA-approved device. Whatever the method, RLT works because you're being exposed to LED (light-emitting diode) light that penetrates deep—between

1 and 2 millimeters into the skin. Mitochondria in your cells absorb this light to make energy and repair themselves. But the levels of light are very low, and don't generate heat, so it should not burn your skin if you follow instructions.

Be sure your skin is clean and makeup free before using. Wear safety goggles to protect your eyes. Each RLT device requires a different time commitment. Some RLT devices need to be used twice a day for thirty to sixty minutes for up to five weeks. Others only take minutes. If you are taking medications that make you sensitive to sunlight, ask your doctor before using.

Rock and Roll to Younger Skin

Facial massage. A 2018 study published in *Complementary Therapies in Medicine* showed that participants who used a facial massage roller for five minutes over a five-week period had improved vasodilation. Better circulation and increased blood flow can improve the appearance of your skin. Massage can also help stimulate lymphatic drainage to drain excess fluids.

A small study published in *PLOS One* in 2017 showed that when you use your favorite go-to antiaging cream in combination with a massage roller, the effects of the cream are more beneficial. Rollers can be made of everything from jade to amethyst to rose quartz. If you want a cooling sensation, your best bet is rose quartz. Pop it in the fridge and you're ready to roll.

Microneedling with a small roller stimulates collagen and elastin production by gently poking the skin. The skin's repair response leads to new cellular growth, and a smoother, tighter, and a brighter complexion. Microneedling can also be done with pen devices, or even topical creams and serums that contain microneedling peptides. Start slow, be gentle, and always clean the device after using. For more dramatic results, see your dermatologist. Participants in a study published in the *Journal of Clinical and Aesthetic Dermatology* (2018) reported an improvement in lines, wrinkles, and skin texture.

Exfoliate with microdermabrasion. Mature skin is usually drier, and dead cells don't slough off as easily, which translates to fine lines, rougher texture, and uneven skin tone. Exfoliation removes those cells and reveals younger, fresher skin underneath. Those new skin cells are better able to hold on to moisture, and they allow other antiaging ingredients to penetrate better and work more effectively.

At-home kits use similar technology to microdermabrasion treatments in a dermatologist's office. The only difference? The exfoliation isn't as deep. Still, regular treatments enhance skin cell turnover and will leave you with softer, smoother skin and fewer fine lines. The most basic products are simply grainy scrubs that you rub on your face with your fingertips.

Follow it up with an antioxidant-rich topical cream. A 2009 study in the *Journal of Dermatological Treatment* found that applying topical antioxidants immediately after professional microdermabrasion increased the number of fibroblasts—cells that produce collagen.

Reveal Younger Skin with Chemical Peels

Mild chemical peels usually rely on AHAs like lactic acid, glycolic acid, or citric acid to exfoliate skin and encourage younger, healthier skin to develop. Unlike microdermabrasion, which physically removes dead skin cells from the skin's top layer, chemical peels dissolve the "glue" that holds cells together so they can slough off. The result is softer, brighter skin with less-noticeable signs of sun damage, such as fine lines, wrinkles, and age spots.

At-home peels use lower concentrations of the acids—typically between 5 and 15 percent, compared to 30 percent for an in-office glycolic acid peel. That means results aren't as dramatic, but with regular use the less-potent treatments are still effective. If you have sensitive skin, you might prefer a peel to microdermabrasion because chemical exfoliation is gentler than manual exfoliation.

Chemical peels work best to reverse the effects of sun damage when they're used along with other antiaging treatments, noted a study in the 2008 issue of *Clinics in Dermatology*. Common combinations include microdermabrasion, Retin-A, and antioxidants. To be safe, check with your dermatologist before using an at-home peel in case any of the ingredients interact with antiaging products you're already using. And as always, you'll need to be diligent about using sunscreen so you don't undo all your results.

Supercharge Your Smile to Look Younger

Your skin is not the only feature to show your age—your smile can give you away too. As you get older, the enamel on your teeth wears away, which can result in chips, yellowing, and stains. Your gums naturally start to recede as well. Around age thirty-five, the elastic tissues around your mouth begin to break down, and the fat that gives volume and plumpness slowly disappears, leading to thinner, flatter lips. You may also notice that the corners of your mouth are starting to droop, and lip lines have begun to form (especially in smokers). Inexpensive lifestyle changes and products can also address many of these telltale signs.

Whiten up. To combat the yellowing and stains that come with age, turn to tooth-whitening products like whitening toothpastes that use mild abrasives or chemicals to remove surface stains. Whitening strips that you can apply at home use hydrogen peroxide to make

---

BRUSH YOUR TEETH GENTLY

Overly vigorous brushing can cause gums to recede faster, so go easy, especially near your gum line. Use a soft-bristled toothbrush and floss at least once daily. Would you like a little high-tech help? Some electric toothbrushes have a two-minute timer and a pressure-sensitive switch that shuts off if you're brushing too hard.

> **LIMIT SUGARY AND ACIDIC FOODS TO PRESERVE YOUR SMILE**
>
> Studies show that snacking on dairy foods, especially cheese, can preserve and even rebuild enamel. But limit sugary and acidic foods and drinks such as soda, fruit juices, coffee, and wine. When you do consume them, brush your teeth or rinse your mouth with water to wash away damaging acids and prevent enamel-eroding plaque and stains from forming.

teeth whiter and brighter. It takes time, but is much cheaper than in-office procedures to whiten teeth. However, whitening strips should only be used in the short term because the hydrogen peroxide can cause sensitivity and can lead to the loss of collagen in the dentin layer of your teeth.

Apply lip gloss. Topical lip plumpers, typically glosses, also offer temporary fullness to thinning lips, usually by irritating sensitive lip skin with stimulants such as mint, pepper, and menthol, and relying on moisturizers to hydrate lips and lend volume. Blue-based red and berry shades of lip color help yellowed teeth appear whiter, but keep it bright, since dark color calls attention to thinning lips. To keep color from migrating, trace lips with liner in the same shade as your lips.

Age-Proof Your Hair

Research shows that after age forty, certain hair cells, called *melanocytes*, exhaust their ability to produce pigment, resulting in graying hair. DNA damage from smoking, sun exposure, and other factors can speed up that process, according to a 2009 study in the journal *Cell*. Hair that gets thinner and weaker with age, and hair loss due to heredity, affects about thirty million American women and fifty million American men beginning as early as age thirty. Here are some tricks to keep your tresses in top shape to instantly look younger.

To dye or not to dye. If you decide to dye, both semipermanent and permanent dyes can add depth and make hair look fuller. But choose your colors carefully. Harsh, one-color dye jobs can age you, so opt for a dye that's within a few shades of your natural color, and add highlights to soften the look.

And if you've been wearing your hair in the same style for the last decade, talk to your stylist about trying out a more modern look that adds volume. Once you hit forty, women should avoid too-long tresses (more than 6 inches [15 cm] past your shoulders) because heavy hair pulls on sagging skin, emphasizing wrinkles.

> **MAKE IT A HABIT: TAKE YEARS OFF YOUR FACE, TEETH, AND HAIR**
>
> **To slow and reverse aging:** Schedule time to try to use at-home therapies, which include RLT, facial massage, microneedling, microdermabrasion, and mild chemical peels.
>
> **Whiten your smile:** Use whitening toothpastes and white strips. Try lip plumpers to improve lip fullness. Avoid too much sugar or foods that are acidic and can damage your teeth.
>
> **Age-proof your hair:** Dye, protect, and moisturize your tresses. Reverse hair loss by boosting circulation and feeding your hair the right nutrients.

Protect your hair from UV rays. Aging hair loses its natural UV defenses as it ages. This can result in sun damage that speeds up the graying process and makes hair brittle and dull. Adding UV protection, especially after you've dyed your hair, can keep hair color from fading.

Restore moisture. Whether you choose to color your salt and pepper strands or not, graying hair is coarser and doesn't reflect light as well. Like the rest of your skin, your scalp produces less oil as you get older. This leads to dry, dull hair that breaks easily. Turn back the clock with moisturizing hair masks and deep conditioners after you color to protect hair and add shine and softness. If you're going gray, choose shampoos and conditioners that prevent yellowing. You may want to shampoo every other day to preserve moisture.

Halt age-related hair loss. If your hair loss is sudden or in a single spot, and you suspect there's another factor involved, like stress or medication side effects, see your dermatologist to determine the cause. For most people, hair loss is hereditary. To help slow it down, focus on nourishing and protecting your roots. First, exercise to boost circulation to your scalp, which stimulates follicles to grow healthy new hair. Next, feed your hair. Hair is made of protein, so load up on protein-rich foods, such as eggs or cottage cheese, to give hair the building blocks it needs.

Biotin, or vitamin B7, forms the basis of hair cells, and a deficiency can cause brittleness or even hair loss. Good sources of B7 include avocados, eggs, milk, nuts, and whole grains. Be gentle with your hair too. You may also want to supplement with up to 5 milligrams of biotin to improve hair growth. Biotin may lower the effects of lipid-lowering medication, so check with your doctor before taking.

Avoid styles that pull on hair—tight rollers, ponytails, weaves, braids, and uncoated rubber bands. They can permanently damage the roots so they can no longer produce hair.

See a Dermatologist to Reduce Signs of Aging

Your dermatologist is a perfect partner as you try to fight the signs of aging skin. Besides having an annual examination to look for skin cancer, you can ask your dermatologist about all kinds of antiaging products, treatments, and procedures, from antioxidant serums (vitamin C and E and more) to lasers, Botox, fillers, and a full-on facelift.

Laser treatments, Botox, and fillers are the most popular in-office treatments. Laser treatments can repair sun damage like fine lines and discoloration, boost collagen production, and improve skin tone and firmness, with a rapid recovery time. Nonablative and fractional lasers work by using heat to damage the dermis, stimulating healing and collagen production while leaving the surrounding skin and the epidermis intact. Both require a series of treatments for best results.

A 2008 study in the *Journal of the American Academy of Dermatology* notes that nonablative lasers work best for treating early signs of aging, while fractional lasers are more effective for moderate wrinkles and sun damage.

Other popular in-office treatments include muscle relaxer, such as Botox, that works best on forehead frown lines, and cosmetic fillers for restoring lost volume to sunken cheeks or thinning lips. Your dermatologist will inject a filler directly into the spot that needs plumping, bulking up the tissue underneath to provide smooth, firm support for skin. The most common fillers are collagen and hyaluronic acid. According to the American Society of Plastic Surgeons, results can last anywhere from two months to a year depending on the type of filler, with certain hyaluronic acid and calcium hydroxylapatite formulas being more likely to hit that yearlong mark. Although soft tissue fillers are generally considered safe, potential side effects include allergic reaction or lumps under the skin.

Permanent fillers such as polymethyl methacrylate (PMMA) may make you look good today, but may not be so flattering down the road. A 2008 study in the *Dermatology Online Journal* also noted that permanent fillers are "less forgiving and less versatile" than temporary fillers, and that people have more complications with permanent fillers, some of which can't be reversed even with surgery. If you opt for fillers of any kind, be sure to find a board-certified dermatologist or plastic surgeon who has experience using injectables, since skill and a good eye are required to use them well.

High-intensity focused ultrasound facial (HIFU) is a new treatment that has yet to gain FDA approval. The 30- to 60-minute procedure relies on ultrasound energy and the heat it generates to target damaged skin tissue. This stimulates the production of collagen to rejuvenate, tighten, and tone the skin and minimize wrinkles without invasive surgery—think facelift. It can be used on the face, neck, eyelids, eyebrows, and chest. Two-thirds of the participants in a 2014 study published in the *Aesthetic Surgery Journal* reported improvement after ninety days of treatment.

Powerful Habits to Turn Back the Clock on Your Body

02

Cultivating strategies to eat well, exercise, reduce stress, and sleep better are essential to staying healthy, strong, and young. How much do you know about the best habits you need to adopt to slow the hands of time?

Test your Body IQ here >

TRUE

FALSE

T F *Adopting the Mediterranean Diet won't do much to reverse aging.*

T F *Eating certain foods generates heat, which burns calories and fat.*

T F *The brain registers liquid calories just as well as those from food.*

T F *Whether you're a man or woman, it's normal for your waistline to expand as you age.*

T F *Getting a good night's sleep can prevent you from piling on the pounds.*

T F *Running is the best aerobic exercise to rev up your metabolism.*

T F *If you don't write down what you're eating and how much you're exercising, it's easy to misjudge whether you're doing enough to lose weight.*

HABIT #1
Feast on Metabolism-Boosting Foods

Eating certain foods generates heat, which burns calories and fat.
TRUE

As your body digests, absorbs, and metabolizes food, it generates body heat—a process called *thermogenesis* that accounts for 10 to 15 percent of your daily calorie expenditure. Certain foods are scientifically proven to increase thermogenesis by small amounts, thereby boosting calorie and fat burn. Making them mainstays in your diet can help you shed unwanted pounds almost effortlessly.

Boost Weight Loss with Ginger

A small 2012 study published in the medical journal *Metabolism* suggests that ginger enhances thermogenesis and reduces feelings of hunger. It may be due to compounds called *gingerols*, which help food digest faster and may stabilize blood sugar levels. Adding a squeeze of lemon to your ginger tea or drinks two or three times a day can also nudge weight loss. That's because the vitamin C in lemon acts as an appetite suppressant. You can also add ginger to a stir-fry made with lean protein and high-fiber veggies like broccoli to take advantage of its antioxidant phytochemical effects.

Rev up Your Metabolism with Spicy Peppers

A 2005 study in the *International Journal of Obesity* found that people ate up to 16 percent fewer calories over the course of two days when they consumed 0.9 grams of ground red pepper (a palatable amount) mixed into tomato juice before each meal. Spicy peppers from the capsicum family contain a compound called *capsaicin,* which gives those peppers their hotness. Around age fifty, you may start to lose taste buds, making flavors duller; spicy foods can help. Studies show that capsaicin can help you shed pounds by spiking your metabolism and helping you eat less overall because it makes you feel full. You eat fiery foods more slowly, giving your brain more time to register that you're full.

Use the Caffeine in Coffee and Green Tea to Burn Calories

Not only does caffeine provide a pick-me-up for flagging energy levels as you get older, but studies show that as little as 50 milligrams can increase thermogenesis by up to 6 percent. Some research shows that epigallocatechin gallate (EGCG) compounds in green tea may make it an even better beverage for weight loss than coffee or other buzz-inducing drinks.

In addition to EGCG's powerful antioxidant effects (which make it an antiaging superstar), a 2010 review of studies in the *American Journal of Clinical Nutrition* showed that, compared with caffeine alone, green tea catechins plus caffeine decreased volunteers' BMIs by 0.55 and boosted weight loss by 3 pounds (1.38 kg).

Not only that, but the combination shrank waistlines by about 0.75 inches (1.93 cm), making it a stellar choice to counteract your body's tendency to deposit fat around your middle as you get older. A 2009 study in the *International Journal of Obesity* found that caffeinated green tea not only helps you drop pounds, but it helps you keep them off as well.

> **MAKE IT A HABIT:**
> **ADD METABOLISM-BOOSTING FOODS**
>
> Add ginger, ground red pepper, and chili peppers to your diet, along with caffeinated drinks like coffee and green tea, to rev up your metabolism. Include fiber-rich foods that take more energy to digest like flaxseed and lentils, which are all protein rich too. Eat lean proteins like chicken, turkey, and fish to build metabolism-maximizing muscle mass.

Take a Green Tea Extract Supplement

If you're not a tea drinker, you can still get green tea's calorie-burning benefits in supplement form: Swiss researchers showed that taking green tea extract with 50 milligrams caffeine and 90 milligrams EGCG at breakfast, lunch, and dinner boosted calorie expenditure by 4 percent over twenty-four hours. That's almost enough to counteract the 5 percent per-decade decrease in metabolism you experience with age.

Pick Protein to Preserve Metabolism-Boosting Muscle

Eating foods that both build muscle and burn calories can help you reverse age-related muscle loss and keep a youthful figure. A 2008 study in the *American Journal of Clinical Nutrition* found that older men and women who consumed 20 percent of total calories from protein lost about 40 percent less muscle than those who ate the least protein (10 percent of their total calories). Protein helps muscles rebuild after exercise, adding muscle mass and increasing strength. It also takes more energy (read: calories) for your body to digest protein than carbs or fat, temporarily boosting your metabolism after you eat. Fish, lean meats, poultry, low-fat dairy, soy foods, legumes, nuts, and seeds are great sources; incorporate protein into each meal or snack for the most muscle-building benefits.

HABIT #2
Escape the Stress-Fat Cycle for a More Youthful Waistline

Whether you're a man or woman, it's normal for your waistline to expand as you age.
TRUE

As you get older, unfortunately, your body naturally starts to deposit more fat around your middle. Men physically have more fat cells in their abdomens, so their bodies prefer to store extra pounds there. For women, declining estrogen levels in midlife signal fat to start accumulating around the waist as well.

Having some fat inside your abdomen is normal, and in fact, it is your body's main source of energy when you face fight-or-flight stress. But long-term—or chronic—stress continually floods your body with high levels of the stress hormone cortisol. That causes you to gain too much belly fat, which in turn raises your risk of cardiovascular disease, high blood pressure, high cholesterol, diabetes, and even cancer.

A 2017 study conducted by the Department of Epidemiology and Public Health at University College London and published in the medical journal *Obesity* showed that participants with higher levels of cortisol over extended periods of time had a higher BMI (body mass index) and a larger waist, and weighed more. But weight gain that results from stress is stubborn and will resist your best efforts at eating healthfully and exercising. To lose your stress fat, especially after age forty, try these tips to become more resilient and put a stop to stress eating.

Beat the Midlife Stress-and-Food Double Whammy

Stress can affect your eating habits in several ways. In 2009, researchers at the University of Michigan found that higher levels of cortisol prompted people to take in more calories and food overall. A 2007 study in the journal *Nutrition* noted that chronic stress makes you

---

MAKE IT A HABIT: STRESS AND BELLY FAT

It's normal for your waistline to expand after age forty. In women, declining estrogen levels lead to greater fat stores at the waist; men have more fat cells there to begin with. Stress adds to belly fat by leading you to overeat, especially with sugary or fatty foods such as cookies and chips. Take control of stress by identifying long-term stressors, relieving tension with noncaloric treats, and taking action to deal directly with issues you're concerned about.

more likely to reach for sugary, fatty foods, possibly because they provide more energy (in the form of calories) to deal with anxiety-inducing events. Sweet, rich foods also activate the release of feel-good chemicals called *endorphins* that act almost like a drug in your system to calm the stress response and improve mood.

But breaking out the brownies can backfire—refined carbs cause a rapid spike and fall in blood sugar, wreaking havoc with insulin levels as they try to restore balance, triggering further cravings and promoting fat storage in your abdomen. With this chain reaction in place, it's no surprise that stress can make you pile on pounds. So, you'll need to add stress management to your diet and exercise regime.

Stress-Proof Your Days for Longer Life (and a Slimmer Figure)

Small changes can make a big difference:

Find a stress relieving meditation. If you feel stressed, stop for a few minutes and tune in to your breath and yourself. You'll be amazed at how quickly stress melts away.

Do a walking meditation. Go outside and focus on your steps and your breath to relax.

Breathe in and out. Inhale slowly through your nose for 1-2-3-4 and exhale through your mouth for 5-6-7-8. Try to let it all go.

Stretch your body. Tension accumulates when we sit too long. Make it a habit to stretch multiple times a day. You can also make it a habit to practice yoga poses like the Extended Triangle, Cat/Cow, and Child's Pose to release tension. Find more poses online.

Stop stressed-out eating. Instead of opting for comfort food, create a list of nonfood feel-better treats, such as buying fresh flowers or getting a massage.

Boost your mood. Put down the doughnut and lace up your sneakers to raise your endorphin levels. Exercise attacks stress fat on both fronts: Not only does it burn calories but also it's a surefire stress reliever. Research shows that even a ten-minute walk can improve your outlook and help you regain perspective.

Taking the initiative to address your stressors is also helpful, since much of our stress comes from feeling like things are out of our control. Try identifying the specific stressor in a situation and picking a response that directly counters it. For example:

Navigating a newly empty nest? Tackle loneliness by blocking out time to connect with friends, current or former coworkers, or a neighbor you've been meaning to introduce yourself to.

Dealing with a sticky family situation? If you're feeling helpless, ask trusted friends for advice and a sense of solidarity.

Planning for retirement got you on edge? If you're concerned about money, make an appointment with a financial advisor to take stock of what you have and set up a budget.

HABIT #3
Lose Weight While You Sleep

Getting a good night's sleep can prevent you from piling on the pounds.
TRUE

Your quality of sleep affects the production of two hormones that control your appetite: ghrelin and leptin. Ghrelin, produced in your gastrointestinal tract, triggers hunger. Leptin is produced in fat cells and tells your brain when you're full. Sleep affects the production of both. A 2024 study in the medical journal *Obesity* showed that sleep deprivation increased levels of ghrelin and lower levels of leptin. This leads to a disruption in the levels of these two important hormones. More ghrelin means you're hungrier and less leptin means your body has trouble signaling that you've had enough, which can lead to overeating.

University of Chicago researchers examined the ghrelin and leptin levels of twelve men after two days of restricted sleep and then two days of extended sleep. Not only did they find that the men's ghrelin levels were higher and leptin levels lower after sleep restriction, making them hungrier, but the men also had cravings for high-calorie, high-carb foods. A 2009 study restricted the sleep of middle-aged men and women to just five-and-a-half hours a night for two weeks. They found that the volunteers took in about 300 more calories from high-carb snacks per day than they did during a two-week period when they slept for eight-and-a-half hours. Even more revealing: Stanford researchers looked at the sleep habits of more than 1,000 people and found that the less sleep they got, the higher their BMI was.

Why Aging Affects Sleep

As you get older, your sleep habits may change. Studies show that circadian rhythms, which manage your sleep/wake cycle, shift with age. That's why even former night owls frequently find themselves going to bed and waking up earlier, spending less time in deep sleep, and sleeping less overall. And according to the National Sleep Foundation, up to 80 percent of older adults with four or more health problems report not sleeping well.

These changes, combined with an increased risk of insomnia and sleep disorders as you get older, can throw off ghrelin and leptin levels, frustrating even the best-laid weight loss plans. Studies also show that estrogen affects ghrelin production, so women in midlife may have an even harder time, thanks to fluctuating hormones.

Sleep, Insulin, and Midlife Obesity

In 2010, researchers at the University of Chicago reviewed studies noting the connection between lack of sleep and obesity. In addition to the ghrelin/leptin link, they found that not getting enough shut-eye can reduce insulin sensitivity. Insulin helps your cells use blood sugar (glucose) for fuel and converts calories into fat. As your body becomes less sensitive, your pancreas has to pump out increasingly greater levels of insulin to make sure your cells get enough glucose and to keep your blood sugar normal.

That extra insulin also means more calories get stored as fat, and as you get older, higher levels of insulin (which is made even worse by sleep deprivation induced cravings for high-carb snacks) makes it more likely that the fat gets stored in your abdomen. Ultimately, this nasty cycle raises your risk for type 2 diabetes, which accelerates aging in almost all of your body's systems.

Snooze to Lose Pounds for Life

Sleep timing, duration, and quality all play a role in keeping your hormones balanced. These guidelines can help:

MAKE IT A HABIT: SLEEP MATTERS

Quality sleep regulates the hormones that trigger hunger and feelings of fullness. Lack of sleep increases cravings for high-carb foods and triggers excess production of insulin, leading to belly fat and possibly diabetes. Sleep problems increase as you get older, so practice good sleep habits to ensure you get enough rest.

Doze off and wake up at approximately the same time every day, including weekends.

Reset your sleep schedule, if you need to. Gradually head to bed fifteen minutes earlier or set your alarm for fifteen minutes later until you've carved out seven or eight hours for sleeping.

Dim the lights. Light signals your brain that it's time to sleep or wake up, so about an hour before bedtime, lower the lights. Keep your bedroom dark at night; purchase light-blocking shades if necessary.

Use a white noise machine. You can choose the sound of rain, thunderstorms, surf, a babbling brook, nature sounds, and more. It can help to block out other noises and soothe you to sleep.

Install a night-light to avoid using the bright overhead light when you take (more frequent) nighttime bathroom breaks. This can make falling back asleep easier.

Check for sleep problems. If you already get enough sleep and still feel tired (and hungry) all the time, ask your doctor if you might have obstructive sleep apnea. Your risk increases as you get older. Apnea can cause you to stop breathing for short periods, sometimes hundreds of times a night. This disrupts your sleep and can leave you feeling groggy during the day, even if you spent eight or nine hours in bed.

HABIT #4
Rev Up Midlife Metabolism, Build Strength, and Improve Flexibility and Balance

Running is the best aerobic exercise to rev up your metabolism.
FALSE

Whether you walk, hike, run, dance, skate, cycle, row, swim, or ski, aerobic activity will help you lose weight and offset the natural decline in metabolism as you get older. Not only do you burn calories during exercise, but your metabolism stays elevated after you finish working out. Exercise can also whittle your waistline, which helps you look younger and will keep you healthy long term. In fact, a 2006 study in the journal *Obesity Reviews* noted that studies using imaging techniques to measure abdominal fat showed that exercise significantly reduced the amount of this particular health-threatening pudge even before subjects saw changes in overall body weight or waist measurements.

As you age, you lose lean muscle mass. And while shedding pounds through diet alone does reduce body fat, it also triggers a further loss of muscle, which ultimately undermines your metabolism. Adding exercise to the equation, however, sets you up for success. Researchers at the University of Pittsburgh School of Medicine found that walking at a moderate intensity three to five times per week for thirty-five to forty-five minutes helped adults in their sixties and early seventies hold on to metabolism-boosting muscle.

Any Exercise Is Better Than No Exercise, But Push Yourself

The National Institute on Aging suggests aiming for at least thirty minutes of moderate-intensity aerobic activity on most or all days of the week, along with flexibility, balance, and strength exercises. If you're new to exercise, talk to your doctor about what kind of activity is best for you and how you can safely start moving and work up to that thirty-minute goal. Any exercise is better than nothing, and as little as ten minutes can stoke your

> **MAKE IT A HABIT: INCREASE EXERCISE**
>
> Amp up your workouts to keep your metabolism high even as you rest. Aim for thirty minutes of moderate-to-vigorous aerobic exercise on most days of the week. Vary your routines to stoke your metabolism and keep you engaged. Shorter exercise routines work too. The important thing is to get moving! Include strength training to build muscle and strength. Stretch three times a week and work to improve your balance.

WEIGHT TRAIN TO REVERSE MUSCLE LOSS

Studies show that previously inactive older adults who start a strength training program can gain up to three pounds of muscle in just three months, boosting metabolism by about 7 percent and muscle strength by 50 percent. To build muscle efficiently, you'll need to do a variety of strength exercises at least twice a week for thirty minutes or more, in addition to doing aerobic exercise for at least thirty minutes on most days of the week. Take at least one day off between strength sessions to let muscles rest and rebuild.

___1 Start with light weights that allow you to perform an exercise with good form (where you can maintain the proper body position and control the weight) at least eight times in a row. If you can't, switch to a lighter weight. If that feels easy to you, trade up to a heavier weight.

___2 For each repetition (rep), focus on making your movements smooth and controlled, taking three seconds to lift, holding for one second, and then taking another three seconds to return to your starting position. Aim for ten to fifteen reps per exercise to make up one set.

___3 Research shows that training with single or multiple sets produces similar strength gains, provided you use a heavy enough weight that you feel fatigued at the end of a set. If you decide to do a single set, you may need to use a slightly heavier weight to reach that point. When doing multiple sets, rest for at least two minutes in between to allow your muscles to refresh their energy resources.

___4 A solid strength-training program includes exercises that address all your major muscle groups: chest, upper and lower back, shoulders and arms, quadriceps (quads) and hips, hamstrings and glutes, calves, and abdominal muscles.

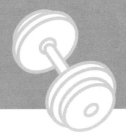

calorie-burning furnace. Still, don't just take a stroll around the block and hang up your sneakers. You'll see more metabolism improvements if you pick up the pace and go a little longer. (Always warm up and cool down with a few minutes of light activity to prevent injury and allow you to push yourself a little harder during your workout.)

Calculate your maximum heart rate by subtracting your age from 220. Exercising vigorously—at about 80 percent of your maximum heart rate—burns the most calories in a session, but check with your doctor to determine a safe range. And duration matters too: If you exercise for more than fifteen minutes, you'll blaze through your body's glycogen stores and start using fat for fuel. Research also shows that working out longer and at a higher intensity keeps your metabolism fired up longer than a shorter, less strenuous sweat session, burning more calories even while you're at rest.

USE NEAT TO FIGHT METABOLISM SLOWDOWN

Your body burns calories performing the necessary functions of living—resting metabolic rate, digesting food, and daily movement—which is scientifically referred to as *activity thermogenesis*. Small bursts of activity throughout the day, or nonexercise activity thermogenesis (NEAT), make up the bulk of the calories you expend and help keep your metabolism fired up. Studies show that NEAT activities can quickly offset the natural decline in your metabolism. Researchers at the Mayo Clinic found people do less NEAT activity as they get older, so intentionally adding it back in can help you stay active, trim, and young. Basically, your goal is to break out of sedentary behaviors, interrupting them with periods of activity.

You can increase your daily NEAT by walking or biking to work or the store instead of driving, pacing or doing chores while you talk or text on the phone, making dinner instead of ordering in, and taking the dog for a walk around the block. If you work at an office, get up for a few minutes every hour to get a drink of water or visit a coworker. Use the stairs instead of the elevator. Deliver news or updates in person rather than email or text. You get the idea—anytime you find yourself sitting, think about how you can make that time more active.

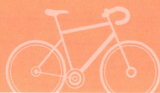

A 2009 study in the journal *Metabolic Syndrome and Related Disorders* found that, in older adults who were not dieting to lose weight, high-intensity exercise (about 75 percent of their aerobic capacity) was more effective than moderate exercise in reducing belly fat. However, if you're also cutting calories to lose weight, moderate-intensity exercise may still do the trick by slimming you down all over, according to a study in the *American Journal of Clinical Nutrition.* In that study, both moderate and vigorous exercise helped subjects preserve muscle during weight loss—a key to keeping your metabolism fired up.

Focus on Flexibility and Core Work to Maintain Balance

As you get older, your muscles become less elastic and tissues around your joints get thicker, which makes movement more difficult. If you don't take action to counteract this, you can lose 10 percent of your flexibility every ten years. Staying flexible can also help you maintain balance and prevent falls, help to relieve chronic pain and tension, and improve circulation, mental focus, and energy. Balance and strength exercises, particularly for your core abdominal muscles and lower body, are key to preventing falls because they give you more control over your body, keep your muscles strong, and improve your coordination. You'll get the most flexibility benefits by purpose-fully stretching your muscles at least three times a week. Keep these steps in mind:

1 *Stretch all your major muscle groups: calves, quadriceps and hamstrings, hip flexors, chest, and lower and upper back. You also can stretch your neck, shoulders, wrists, and ankles. Always warm up first, since stretching a cold muscle can raise your risk of pulling it.*

2 *Don't force the stretch or bounce, but slowly and smoothly ease into the stretch, keeping your joints slightly bent, and hold it for at least thirty seconds. Breathe normally throughout. Repeat each stretch three to five times, and try to reach a little further each time. You might feel a little discomfort as you extend your reach, but you should stop if you feel pain.*

3 *Stretch periodically throughout the day if that makes it easier to fit it in, or you can set aside a block of time to stretch your whole body. Exercises like yoga, Pilates, tai chi, and resistance stretching combine multiple benefits of flexibility, balance, and strength.*

EXERCISE AND MORE TRACKER

Aim for at least thirty minutes of moderate-intensity aerobic activity on most or all days of the week, along with strength, balance, and flexibility exercises. Don't forget to include NEAT too. Daily activities like biking to work, walking the dog, or taking the stairs keep you moving!

Su
STRENGTH

BALANCE

FLEXIBILITY

Mo
STRENGTH

BALANCE

FLEXIBILITY

Tu
STRENGTH

BALANCE

FLEXIBILITY

We
STRENGTH

BALANCE

FLEXIBILITY

Th
STRENGTH

BALANCE

FLEXIBILITY

Fr
STRENGTH

BALANCE

FLEXIBILITY

Sa
STRENGTH

BALANCE

FLEXIBILITY

Variety Is the Spice of Exercise

To keep your metabolism humming, variety is critical. Modify your exercise routine from time to time to challenge new muscles, or add in a few sprintlike bursts of activity to burn more calories and fat without feeling like you're working harder overall. You can alter the length of your workouts as well, which not only helps you fit in exercise when you have time, but also allows you to focus on different benefits. An intense twenty-minute workout will torch calories, for instance, while a long, steady workout boosts endurance and burns more fat. Variety also helps you beat boredom and reduces your risk of injury, ensuring that you can stay active.

BUILD BALANCE TO AGE WELL

You can do balance exercises just about anywhere, but when you start, make sure you have a wall or chair nearby in case you become unsteady. The National Institute on Aging recommends basic balance exercises such as standing on one foot, walking heel to toe, and walking with slow, exaggerated steps in a straight line with your arms stretched out to your sides. Engaging small muscles in your abdominal core will keep you upright and steady.

Try standing up from a seated position without using your hands, one-legged squats, and many upper-body exercises (like biceps curls) while standing on one foot. You can also use balance pads, boards, and discs to improve your balance. Exercises like crunches, squats, and push-ups are good too, because they engage your core, challenge your muscles in new ways, and make you work harder to maintain balance.

Powerful Habits to Turn Back the Clock on Your Brain

03

Aging is a fact of life, but there are many ways that you can protect your brain. Adopting healthy habits can ensure your noggin is in great shape for years to come.

Test your Brain IQ >

TRUE

FALSE

T F *Inflammation plays a role in age-related cognitive decline, stroke, and Parkinson's disease.*

T F *Chronic health conditions have no impact on cognitive health.*

T F *Aging can make you more prone to depression, which can cause stress, trigger pain, aggravate chronic conditions, and age your brain.*

T F *Once you begin to lose your memory, it's very difficult to change the neural pathways and strengthen your brain.*

T F *Your brain is hardwired and as you age it becomes more difficult to improve its function.*

T F *Cognitive decline and age-related diseases like Alzheimer's result from free radical damage in the brain.*

HABIT #1
Eat a Diet to Cool Inflammation and Keep Your Brain Young

Inflammation plays a role in age-related cognitive decline, stroke, and Parkinson's disease.
TRUE

Inflammation is a factor in many chronic diseases, including dementia, Alzheimer's, and other neurodegenerative conditions. The good news is that research shows you can do a lot to keep your brain healthy and young—including eating an anti-inflammatory diet.

Mediterranean Diet Fights Inflammation

Dining on foods rich in antioxidants, healthy fats, and whole grains, and avoiding foods that trigger inflammation, such as saturated and trans fats and refined carbs, help keep your brain in top shape. This way of eating, as exemplified in the Mediterranean diet, has been shown to reduce the risk of Alzheimer's and vascular dementia. Another benefit: It can help you stay at a healthy weight, which reduces the risk of dementia.

Learn to Love Fruits and Veggies

Fruits and vegetables are fantastic sources of antioxidants, vitamins, minerals, fiber, and other anti-inflammatory compounds called *phytonutrients* that help keep your brain young. Antioxidants fight free radicals that damage cells and trigger inflammation. Folate, found in broccoli, lentils and beans, spinach, and asparagus, helps keep brain synapses firing correctly. Thousands of phytonutrients in plant foods exert all kinds of beneficial brain effects, including mopping up free radicals. Aim for five to nine servings a day.

Eat Healthy Fats to Keep Your Brain in Top Shape

Omega-3s create hormones that dampen inflammation throughout your body—including your brain. They also thin your blood slightly, making it easier for your brain to get the oxygen-rich blood it needs to function optimally. A 2023 study in *The American Journal of Clinical Nutrition* showed that eating foods high in omega-3s or long-term supplementation of this healthy fat can reduce the risk of dementia or cognitive decline by 20 percent. Fatty, cold-water fish, like salmon, mackerel, anchovies, sardines, and herring (think: SMASH), as well as lake trout, are the best sources. Grass-fed beef, fortified foods (like eggs), walnuts, ground flaxseed, and soy foods like tofu contain omega-3s as well. Broccoli, cabbage, and other leafy greens supply small amounts.

> **MAKE IT A HABIT:**
> **ANTI-INFLAMMATORY DIET BASICS**
>
> Eat five to nine servings of fruits and vegetables per day. Eat two servings per week of fish high in omega-3 fats: Think SMASH: salmon, mackerel, anchovies, sardines, and herring, along with lake trout. Eat three servings of whole grains per day. Exercise to improve brain function and keep chronic diseases away.

Eat "Superfoods" to Stay Sharp as You Age

Superfoods contain antioxidants that boost memory, slow brain aging, and protect against Antioxidants are critical for brain health because they fight free radicals, which can interfere with how your brain cells process nutrients, cause oxidative damage that can lead to cell death, and keep brain cells from communicating with each other, leading to memory loss.

Color is one indication of which phytonutrients a plant contains, so eating a variety of brightly colored fruits and vegetables is the best way to ensure you get broad-spectrum protection against oxidative stress. Go organic if you can to avoid pesticides and other contaminants. Keep your brain young with these foods:

Blueberries contain a number of polyphenols, including anthocyanins—water-soluble antioxidants—that give fruits and vegetables a red or purple color and can improve cognitive function and memory. A 2010 study in the *Journal of Agricultural and Food Chemistry* found that older adults with mild memory problems who drank wild blueberry juice every day for twelve weeks showed improved scores on memory tests. Blackberries, raspberries, cherries, red grapes, pomegranates, red cabbage, and beets are also good sources of anthocyanins.

Dark leafy greens like kale, spinach, and collards can be a source of many brain-boosting nutrients like magnesium. The darker green, the better, which means iceberg lettuce doesn't count. Greens also contain antioxidants like chlorophyll to quench free radicals. According to a 2018 study in *Neurology*, just one serving of leafy greens a day can help keep the brain young and ward off cognitive decline. Researchers think it's because of the plant-based compounds in greens, which include phylloquinone, folate, and lutein. Make a salad and sprinkle antioxidant and omega-3-rich walnuts and flax-seeds on top to further boost brain health.

Curcumin is the component of the curry spice turmeric responsible for its yellow color, and appears to protect the brain in at least ten different ways. For one, it defends the brain against stress-induced memory problems, according to a 2009 study in the journal *Neuropharmacology*. When it comes to Alzheimer's, studies show it improves memory by delaying the breakdown of neurons, decreasing plaque formation, removing toxic metals like cadmium and lead, calming inflammation, and fighting free radicals. Eat Indian curries, and add a teaspoon of turmeric to soups, rice dishes, sauces, marinades, or even to scrambled eggs. Add black pepper and healthy fats to improve absorption.

Grapes and red wine. Like blueberries, anthocyanins give red grapes their color. A 2009 study in the *British Journal of Nutrition* found that the juice improved cognitive function in adults with early memory problems. Red wine contains high concentrations of another superstar antioxidant: resveratrol. This antioxidant protects against age-related cognitive decline and according to a 2009 study in the *European Journal of Pharmacology*. Limit yourself to two glasses of red wine a week for women and three for men. Drink Concord grape juice to protect against Alzheimer's plaques and calm inflammation.

Galangal and ginger. Galangal is found in southern Asia, has been used in Ayurvedic medicine, and is a close relative of ginger and turmeric. All are rich in plant-based antioxidants known as *polyphenols* that fight free radical damage and may improve memory. You can eat ginger and galangal fresh (check your local Asian market) or include these antioxidant powerhouses in recipes for Chinese and Thai dishes.

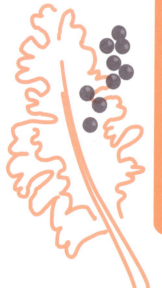

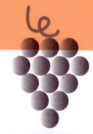

GO ORGANIC!

Eating organic produce and other foods with the United States Department of Agriculture (USDA) Organic label as often as you can is a smart move. That's because chronic low-dose exposure to organophosphorus pesticides (the most commonly used pesticides in the United States) results in cognitive impairment. Pesticides also age your brain by triggering inflammation and increasing damaging free radicals. You'll find an annually updated list of the dirty dozen, the foods highest in pesticides, at the Environmental Working Group website. It commonly includes strawberries, pears, apples, grapes, cherries, peaches, and spinach.

Eat More Whole Grains to Slow Brain Aging

Whole grains contain fiber, which can scrub damaging plaques from your brain arteries. They also boast antioxidants and nutrients, like thiamin, that calm inflammation. Refined carbohydrates and sweets, on the other hand, spike your blood sugar and trigger inflammation. High blood sugar (anything over 100 mg/dL, the cutoff point for prediabetes) increases your risk of stroke. And research shows that excess insulin—produced in response to high blood sugar—accelerates brain aging and increases risk of cognitive impairment and dementia, including Alzheimer's disease.

To keep your blood sugar steady, eat three servings of whole grains per day (half of your total grain intake). Your best bet is to eat actual whole grains, rather than whole-grain flours and products, which have been processed to remove some of the beneficial parts of the grain. Barley, oats (especially steel-cut), quinoa, millet, wheat berries, and brown rice are all good choices.

HABIT #2
Manage Depression and Stress to Minimize Brain Aging

Aging can make you more prone to depression, which can cause stress, trigger pain, aggravate chronic conditions, and age your brain.
TRUE

The areas of the brain responsible for learning, memory, higher-level thinking, and decision making—the medial temporal lobe (hippocampus) and prefrontal cortex—are susceptible to depression and stress, which can amplify age-related cognitive decline. Thankfully, you can keep your brain young and healthy by adopting lifestyle changes that protect against depression and stress.

The Problem with Depression and Aging

Evidence, including a 2010 study in the journal *Psychiatry Research*, suggests that major depressive disorder can have harmful and lasting effects on cognitive function. A 2010 study in the *British Journal of Psychiatry* did brain scans on people over the age of sixty who had major depression and found that cognitive deficits due to depression most likely stem from blood vessel damage in the brain.

Depression especially affects your ability to understand language and process information quickly, making you feel fuzzy-headed, according to a 2010 study in *Neuropsychobiology*. And mild depression can trigger brain changes as well, so even if you're just feeling a little blue, it's worth taking steps to deal with the depression before it does too much damage.

Get Moving

Whether you are depressed, think you might be, or are concerned about keeping depression at bay as you get older, your first step is to talk to your doctor about lifestyle changes that can protect against depression and even help lift it. For example, countless studies demonstrate exercise's ability to stimulate endorphins, those feel-good neurotransmitters, and boost mood.

A 2006 study by Canadian researchers suggests that exercise might also alleviate depression by stimulating new neurons. Exercise can help you hang on to functional ability longer as well, allowing you to stay active, live independently, and maintain social connections—all of which can help you ward off depression. If these strategies don't suffice, talk to your doctor about medications that might help. Be sure to discuss potential side effects, since those can significantly affect your quality of life.

EXERCISE TO KEEP YOUR BRAIN FIT FOR LIFE

In addition to eating well, a 2009 study in the journal *The Physician and Sportsmedicine* notes that exercise promotes the creation of new neurons, increases brain volume, and improves cognitive function—all of which help aging brains retain plasticity, or the ability to create new neural connections. Exercise increases the number of neurons, improves their responsiveness, and regulates important neurotransmitters responsible for cell communication, helping you stay sharp. Regular exercise may also delay the onset of dementia and Alzheimer's disease, reported researchers in a 2006 study in the *Annals of Internal Medicine*. Exercise also boosts oxygen-rich blood flow to your brain.

A 2014 study in the *British Journal of Sports Medicine* showed that regular aerobic exercise helped to increase the volume of the hippocampus, the part of the brain that's responsible for learning and memory in women with probable mild cognitive impairment. Aim for at least thirty minutes of moderate aerobic exercise on most (or all) days of the week. Exercising outdoors may boost brain health even more, suggests a 2008 study in the journal *Psychological Science*. Researchers found that people who walked in natural environments performed better on memory and attention tests than those exercising in urban settings. Strength training and even daily activities help improve cognitive function as well.

Set Up Social Support to Age Well and Ward Off Depression

As you get older, your natural points of connection with others change and often diminish. If you don't take steps to maintain existing relationships and create new ones, a sense of isolation can creep in, bringing with it a higher risk of depression and cognitive decline. The second half of life brings with it opportunities to deepen friendships and expand your social circle. Plenty of research shows the brain benefits of a strong social network. The landmark MacArthur Foundation study found that maintaining social and intellectual connections was one of the most significant characteristics of successful aging among the more than 1,000 adults who participated in the study.

A 2008 study in the *American Journal of Public Health* suggested that larger social networks protect cognitive function. An active social life, along with mental and physical activity, leads to improved cognition and protects against dementia, according to a 2004 study in *Lancet Neurology.*

The number, frequency, and degree of interactions with others all factor in, and all kinds of links—from waving at a neighbor to sharing deep concerns with a trusted friend—are included. Meeting people can forge new neural connections, and interacting with others activates several areas of your brain.

> **MAKE IT A HABIT: MANAGE DEPRESSION AND STRESS**
>
> Spend time in nature to relieve stress and improve mood. Walk in a forest, in the mountains, or on the beach. Exercise to lift your mood; even ten minutes can relieve the blues. Stay socially connected; isolation worsens depression, which results in foggy thinking. Reduce stress by taking deep breaths. Keep a calendar and lists to manage your busy life and help you make decisions.

To find new friends, try something new, take a yoga class, join a book club, volunteer, go back to school, or sign up for group travel. Bring a friend along to make it easier to step out of your comfort zone. Walking or running clubs, exercise classes, group hikes, or playing a few rounds of golf with friends are all excellent ways to get fit and expand your social circle at the same time. Combining social and intellectual pursuits is another way to meet people and stay sharp. Start a chess club, attend a lecture, teach a class, or volunteer to tutor in your local schools.

Stop Stress in Its Tracks for Lifelong Brainpower

Moderate amounts of stress hormones can actually improve cognitive function and memory, but exposing your brain to too much for too long can mess with your mind. The hippocampus, the area of your brain responsible for long-term memory and spatial navigation, has more glucocorticoid receptors (for stress hormones, such as cortisol) than other parts of the brain, making it more vulnerable to chronic

> **NATURE CURE**
>
> If you feel stressed or depressed, go outside and take a walk in the forest. Research led by Dr. Qing Li at the Nippon Medical School in Japan has shown forest bathing, or *shinrin-yoku*, reduces stress, improves memory and concentration, and boosts energy among other benefits. This is in part thanks to the composition of the oxygen-rich forest air and the fact that the chemicals expelled by trees to fight diseases actually boost human immunity. Forests with high levels of humidity are also full of negative ions. A 2018 review of studies on ionization show that exposure to negative ions relieves stress, regulates mood, and improves immune function. You can also take advantage of this effect by taking a stroll on the beach because negative ions are created when water collides with itself. Walking in the mountains after a thunderstorm (ions persist after a storm has passed) and near waterfalls also offers exposure to negative ions. Indoors, ionizers, and Himalayan salt lamps provide benefits too.

stress. As you get older, your hippocampus undergoes changes—such as losing synapses and having them become less responsive—and adding stress to the picture accelerates that brain aging, affecting memory and your speed of processing information. Stress hormones may also kill brain cells and shrink your hippocampus.

Keeping anxiety in check appears to undo stress-related damage and helps keep your brain working at its best. A 2010 study in the *Journal of Neuroscience* noted that counteracting cortisol restores spatial memory, keeps synapses adaptable to taking in new experiences (called plasticity, which is the basis for learning and memory and typically declines with age), and helps neurons in your hippocampus fire properly. Simple strategies like these can help you subdue stress, relieve depression, and get your brain back.

Take a slow, deep breath with a longer exhale than your inhale. Try breathing in for 1-2-3-4 and exhale for 5-6-7-8 through the mouth. Often, people breathe shallowly when stressed, and lack of oxygen for the brain can affect your memory and damage your hippocampus.

Do simple yoga stretches. Yoga improves flexibility and balance, and stretching relieves stress. Try poses like Extended Triangle, Downward Dog, Cat/Cow, and Child's Pose.

Build a social network to turn to in difficult times.

Try keeping a calendar or to-do list to stay focused. Decision making and planning are use-it-or-lose-it components of cognitive health, and having a plan for the day can help you feel more in control.

Sleep Deprivation = Depression

Older adults are more likely to experience both depression and sleep problems. Improving sleep or treating depression can benefit both conditions and lead to better brain function. It may also help maintain cognitive function in older adults.

If you have a chronic sleep problem, like insomnia, restless legs syndrome, or obstructive sleep apnea (all of which are more common as you get older), talk to your doctor or a sleep specialist to design a treatment plan. Certain health conditions or medications may trigger sleep problems as well; work with your doctor to get health issues under control or switch medicines if needed. If health problems aren't interfering with your sleep, there are some easy ways to ensure a good night's rest:

- *Start by determining how much sleep you actually need. Most people over fifty require between seven and nine hours a night.*

- *Try going to bed at a consistent time and letting yourself wake up naturally without an alarm for a full week, without napping during the day if possible. Once you know how much you need, you may find you have to alter your bedtime routine in order to get the full amount.*

- *Lifestyle changes like setting a regular sleep schedule and keeping your bedroom dark can help you fall and stay asleep.*

- *If you need help getting drowsy for an earlier bedtime, about an hour beforehand, dim the lights and switch to quieter activities, like reading a lighthearted book or meditating.*

- *Taking a hot bath or shower before bed also helps by raising your core body temperature—once you're out of the hot water, the resulting temperature drop allows you to fall asleep faster and sleep more soundly.*

- *Avoid drinking alcohol or consuming caffeine for three to four hours before bed, and if you still have trouble sleeping, cut them out completely.*

- *If an overactive mind is keeping you awake, stash a notebook on your nightstand to write down concerns or tomorrow's to-do list and try a mind-body technique like progressive muscle relaxation to help quiet your mind.*

- *If you've tried all these lifestyle changes and are still having trouble sleeping, consider taking melatonin or another natural remedy.*

- *Prescription sleep aids can also be effective, but they carry greater risks of potentially serious side effects and may be habit forming—use them as a last resort.*

HABIT #3
Sharpen Mental Focus with Mind-Body Techniques

Once you begin to lose your memory, it's very difficult to change the neural pathways and strengthen your brain.

FALSE

There are many mind-body practices that you can make a habit to help you regain focus and stay sharp. More than just memory tricks, these techniques can actually change neural pathways and strengthen your mental muscle. Put them into practice now to reap immediate brain benefits; they're even more effective the longer you do them.

Make Meditation a Habit to Maintain Your Mental Acuity

More people are meditating than ever before. In fact, between 2002 and 2022, the number has doubled from 7.5 to 17.3 percent, according to The National Health Interview Survey. Although researchers aren't sure yet just how meditation protects against age-related cognitive decline and dementia, mounting evidence suggests it can slow brain aging in a number of ways.

For example, meditation can relieve memory-sapping stress and prevent oxidative damage from free radicals, and it may also strengthen brain cell circuits and communication and offset age-related shrinking of your brain's cerebral cortex (the area that controls memory, language, and sensory processing). A 2017 study in *Scientific Reports* conducted with long-time expert meditators suggests that, over time, meditation may reduce age-related structural and functional brain changes. In broad terms, there are two main forms of meditation:

Focused attention meditation means concentrating on an object, a word, your breath, or another element for a sustained period.

Open monitoring, or mindfulness meditation, involves being present in the moment to evaluate experiences without reacting to or judging them, helping you to recognize patterns of emotion and thought. A 2006 study in *Nature Neuroscience* found that lapses in attention result from reduced activity in the parts of your brain responsible for concentration, which leads to less efficient processing of the situation at hand.

However, researchers noted in a 2008 review of studies that several aspects of attention can be learned, such as detecting and disengaging from distraction and redirecting your attention back to your original point of focus. They concluded that focused-attention meditation can help you hone those skills. Research also shows that this type of meditation can boost blood flow to the brain, bringing oxygen and glucose needed for energy and optimal functioning.

Mindfulness or open-monitoring meditation may help synchronize neuron firing, an important feature of synapse "plasticity" (or adaptability), which is the basis for learning and memory, and typically declines with age. It can also help increase your ability to focus. More studies are needed to determine which kind of meditation has the biggest brain benefits, whether there are important common elements in the different kinds, and what "dose" you need to reap the most mental gains, but as little as ten minutes a day can make a difference. Working up to thirty to forty minutes a day may bring additional benefits.

Perhaps the most common types are transcendental meditation (a form of focused attention meditation using a mantra) and mindfulness meditation (open monitoring, involving being mindful of your surroundings or experience). Most forms involve sitting still in a quiet place, but if you find it difficult to quiet your thoughts while staying stationary, try a walking meditation (brain bonus: exercise!).

> **MAKE IT A HABIT:**
> **MIND-BODY RELAXATION**
>
> Meditate for ten minutes a day, working up to thirty minutes. Do yoga or a walking meditation to reap the combined mental benefits of stress reduction and exercise. Pray and regularly attend religious services to reduce cognitive decline.

Use Mind-Body Approaches to Relax and Retrain Your Brain

Yoga, yoga Nidra (yogic sleep), guided imagery and visualization, prayer, and progressive muscle relaxation are other mind-body techniques you can use to boost brain health. Their main benefit is stress reduction, but they offer other mental advantages as well. Yoga, for instance, also increases circulation to bring oxygen-rich blood to the brain.

Guided imagery—forming mental pictures about relaxing places or situations—stimulates your imagination and senses, and a 2004 study in *Psychological Reports* indicates that it can also improve working memory (responsible for helping you hold on to recently learned bits of information). Other research on guided imagery suggests that being more relaxed can help you process information better.

Prayer shares similarities with meditation, and a 2009 study in the *Journals of Gerontology: Biological Sciences and Medical Sciences* further noted that regularly attending religious services is associated with a lower risk of cognitive decline.

Finally, progressive muscle relaxation, which involves slowly tightening and relaxing muscles starting at your toes or head and moving up or down the body, respectively, helps you let go of tension in your body and mind, preparing you to learn and remember information more easily.

HABIT #4
Challenge Your Brain to Improve Cognition as You Get Older

Your brain is hardwired, and as you age, it becomes more difficult to improve its function.
FALSE

Your brain circuitry is not hardwired—it's actually quite adaptable. The scientific term is *neuroplasticity,* and although it decreases with age, your adult brain retains a significant capacity to modify itself based on your experiences and how you interact with your environment. Neuroplasticity is considered the basis for learning and memory, and losing it can lead to age-related cognitive decline. But consistently challenging your brain and exposing yourself to new people, places, and experiences can form new brain cells, strengthen neural connections so you can store and retrieve information more easily, and keep your brain young.

Break Out of a Rut to Grow New Brain Cells

Studies show that novelty boosts neural responses. A 2020 study showed that novelty also boosts the production of the neurotransmitter dopamine, which makes learning easier. This means doing the same job, going to the same places, and doing the same things won't do much to keep you cognitively active. One way to work novelty into your life is through leisure activities. In one *New England Journal of Medicine* study, people over seventy-five who participated in hobbies such as reading, playing board games, playing musical instruments, and dancing reduced their risk of dementia.

For the best brain benefits, try something you haven't done before, or at least attempt a variation on the theme. If you enjoy swing dancing, give the tango a twirl. Loved learning French? Use that dopamine rush to pick up Spanish or Italian more easily. If you play the piano, put down classical music for a while and try your hand at jazz or blues.

Changing your environment can also engage your brain by challenging your visual and spatial memory and stimulating your senses. It can be as dramatic as rearranging your furniture and painting your walls a new color, or as minor as organizing your drawers differently and growing some fragrant herbs. You can also try taking a new route to familiar places like the grocery store, try a new restaurant, or visit a new city or country.

Go Beyond Crossword Puzzles to Boost Your Brainpower

Online word games, crosswords, sudoku, and other puzzles and memory exercises can be mentally stimulating, and research shows they're great additions to your brain-boosting toolkit. A 2002 study in the *Journal of the American Medical Association* followed a group of 800 adults over the age of sixty-five to see how participating in stimulating activities protected cognitive function. They found that people who did activities that involved processing information—such as watching TV; listening to the radio; reading newspapers, magazines, and books; playing games such as cards, checkers, crosswords, or other puzzles; and going to museums—nearly every day reduced their risk of developing Alzheimer's disease by almost 50 percent.

You can also use technology to challenge your brain. For example, a 2009 study in the *American Journal of Geriatric Psychiatry* found that searching the internet increases brain activity, especially in the areas of decision making and complex reasoning. Playing online brain-teasing video games give your gray matter a workout and stimulate your mind. Some games reduce anxiety by teaching your brain to focus on the positive, rather than the negative.

As powerfully protective as these activities are, however, they don't offer social connection or physical activity, two other important tenets of brain health. You'll have an even better brain benefit if you can combine some aspects of intellectual, physical, and social stimulation.

If you'd like to learn knitting, quilting, or painting, see if a local yarn shop or craft store offers group classes. Interested in learning something new? Go to lectures at a local community center, a college, a wildlife rescue center, or the zoo. Volunteer to walk and play with pets at an animal adoption center. If you love to read, see if a local bookstore holds author signings or discussion groups. Invite a friend to explore a walking or hiking path in a different neighborhood or play pickleball with you.

> **MAKE IT A HABIT: BRAIN BOOSTERS**
>
> Do something different in your daily routine: Take a new route home, try a twist on your hobby, or eat at a new restaurant. Use technology to stimulate your brain. Search the web for things you're interested in or play a video game. Combine mentally stimulating activities with social interactions or exercise to double the brain benefits.

HABIT #5
Tap Antioxidant Supplements and More to Boost Brain Health

Cognitive decline and age-related diseases like Alzheimer's result from free radical damage in the brain.
TRUE

A growing body of research suggests that cognitive decline and age-related diseases like Alzheimer's result from free radical damage in the brain. So, it makes sense to tap the power of antioxidants in supplements like vitamins C and E, which are proven free radical fighters and work synergistically to protect cells from oxidative damage. Because vitamin E is fat soluble, it has access to parts of the brain (which is more than 60 percent fat) that other antioxidants can't reach, making it especially valuable.

A 2004 study in the journal *Archives of Neurology* found that older adults who took 500 milligrams of vitamin C and 400 IU of vitamin E supplements together had lower risk of developing Alzheimer's disease. If you supplement with vitamin E, look for mixed natural tocopherols or d-alpha tocopherol rather than the synthetic form, dl-alpha tocopherol.

WHY THE BRAIN NEEDS B12

Vitamin B12 is not an antioxidant but it's worth adding to improve cognition. A 2020 study in the medical journal *Cureus* concluded that a B12 deficiency is linked to cognitive decline. B12 also plays a role in building myelin, the protein and fatty sheath that encases the nervous system in the brain and spinal cord. B12 may also help oxygenate brain cells and cool inflammation. The recommended daily allowances (RDAs) for vitamin B12 is 2.4 micrograms, or take a quality multivitamin that contains B12. According to NIH, supplements offer 50 percent more bioavailability than foods sources like meat, fish, or dairy products.

> **MAKE IT A HABIT:**
> **SUPPLEMENTS AND MORE FOR BRAIN HEALTH**
>
> Take 500 milligrams of vitamin C and 400 IU of vitamin E supplements daily, and ask your doctor about adding a nonsteroidal antiinflammatory drug (NSAID) four times a week. With vitamin E, look for mixed natural tocopherols or d-alpha tocopherol rather than the synthetic form, dl-alpha tocopherol. Take coenzyme Q10 (CoQ10) to fight free radicals in the brain. Take 2.4 micrograms of B12 daily to improve cognition. Try 120 milligrams of ginkgo biloba once or twice a day to preserve, and possibly improve, long-term memory and cognitive function.

Coenzyme Q10 (CoQ10) is another fat-soluble antioxidant able to get into fatty brain cell membranes and protect them from free radicals. It's made by every cell in your body and helps the mitochondria—cell structures responsible for producing energy—do their job. With aging, however, levels of CoQ10 decline, and your brain may not have enough to perform all of its critical functions or to protect itself against free radicals. Preliminary studies show encouraging results with supplementing for Alzheimer's and especially Parkinson's disease, but more research in humans is needed. For basic brain health, start with 30 milligrams a day.

Herbs for Clearer Thinking

Ginkgo biloba is possibly the best-known supplement for brain health. Ginkgo contains antioxidant compounds called flavonoids and terpenoids that can help prevent free radical damage to the brain that might impair mental function. It also increases blood flow to the brain, potentially enhancing memory. Phytochemicals in gingko may also act as antioxidants to protect nerve cells from free radical damage. There is plenty of promising research on the herb not just for preventing cognitive decline but also for improving existing dementia and Alzheimer's.

For example, a 2010 review of studies in the journal *Pharmacopsychiatry* found that using standardized ginkgo biloba extract for six months improved cognitive function in people with dementia. And a 2009 review of studies in *Human Psychopharmacology* noted that consistently taking ginkgo improves higher-level thinking and long-term memory.

Powerful Habits to Turn Back the Clock on Your Bones and Joints

04

As you age, your bones and joints deserve special attention. The good news is, there is much that you can do to ensure strong bones and flexible joints starting today.

Test your Bones and Joints IQ >

TRUE

FALSE

(T) (F) *As you get older, you lose bone faster than you can regrow it (up to 1 percent per year after age thirty-five).*

(T) (F) *Whether you're underweight or overweight, it doesn't affect your joints.*

(T) (F) *Drinking milk is the only way to build strong bones.*

(T) (F) *It's not enough to eat a diet rich in vitamins and minerals like calcium and vitamin D; it's also important to avoid diet don'ts.*

(T) (F) *Natural remedies can be a helpful adjunct and are often safer than some conventional treatments and therapies for joint and bone health.*

(T) (F) *Alternative therapies are just woo-woo approaches that have little effect on bone and joint health.*

(T) (F) *Joint pain can become worse if it's left untreated.*

HABIT #1
Achieve and Keep a Healthy Weight to Reduce Joint Stress and Protect Your Bones

Whether you're underweight or overweight, it doesn't affect your joints.
FALSE

Being underweight increases your risk of osteoporosis and fracture. Being overweight increases the pressure on your joints. Staying within the normal weight range for your height is one of the best things you can do to protect your body against all kinds of age-related health problems, including cognitive decline and heart disease. Your weight also affects your body mechanically (pressure on joints, effort required to move your limbs, etc.) and chemically (levels of circulating hormones, neurotransmitters, and other substances). So getting to—and staying at—a healthy weight is key to keeping all of your body systems in balance. And research shows it can also benefit your bones and joints.

Gain Weight by Adding Muscle Mass to Keep Bones Strong

Being underweight increases your risk of osteoporosis and fracture. A 2023 study in *Scientific Reports* conducted in Korea showed that in that population being underweight and over forty was a risk for fractures, even if someone returned to a normal weight. Another study with over 100,000 people published in *Scientific Reports* in 2024 showed a relationship between a low BMI and the risk of osteoporosis. The authors noted, "These findings highlight the importance of maintaining normal weight for optimal bone health."

An earlier 2010 study in the *Archives of Gerontology and Geriatrics* found that postmenopausal women who had a lower BMI and sarcopenia (age-related muscle loss) had correspondingly lower bone mineral content and density, possibly raising their risk of fracture. If you need to gain weight, you'll get the best bone and joint benefits by adding pounds of muscle rather than fat. Increasing muscle strength and control stimulates bone growth and helps stabilize your bones and joints to protect you from falls.

Calculate Your Resting Metabolic Rate

To gain 1 pound (454 g) of fat, you'll need to add roughly 3,500 calories to your diet. If you step up your strength training to boost muscle, you may need to eat more, since muscle burns more calories than fat. It may be tempting to turn to foods high in fat and refined carbs, like cake and croissants, to increase calorie intake, but that approach will ultimately backfire by harming other aspects of your health. Instead, fill your plate with healthful higher-calorie foods that provide valuable nutrients, such as avocados, nuts, and olive oil. Protein-rich foods will also help you build and maintain muscle.

A regular regimen of strength training exercises that uses weights, elastic bands, or your own body weight for resistance is the best way to add muscle and ensure that the extra calories you take in don't convert to fat. Studies show that a strength training program can help you gain up to 3 pounds (1.4 kg) of muscle in just three months. Ask your doctor which strength training moves will help you safely and effectively put on muscle while protecting your bones and joints.

Lose Weight to Lighten the Load on Aging Joints

Being overweight increases the stress on your joints—each extra 1 pound (455 g) of weight you carry puts another 3 to 4 pounds (1.4–1.8 kg) of pressure on your knees and hips because of the extra force exerted when your foot hits the ground. This worsens pain, stiffness, and range of movement. Research shows that people with higher BMIs also tend to change their gait, walking more slowly and exerting greater impact forces because of the changes to their stride. But losing even a few pounds can relieve some of the burden on those hardworking hinges. A 2005 study in *Osteoarthritis and Cartilage* found that overweight and obese adults with knee osteoarthritis who lost 10 percent of their body weight increased their knee function by almost 30 percent.

> **MAKE IT A HABIT:**
> **REACH AND MAINTAIN A HEALTHY WEIGHT**
>
> If you need to gain weight to stave off osteoporosis, choose quality calories such as fruits and vegetables, nuts and seeds, and healthy fats—not cake. Combine a weight-gain program with strength training to ensure the extra calories don't get stored as fat. If you need to shed extra pounds by eating less, avoid losing bone mass by increasing your calcium and protein intake.

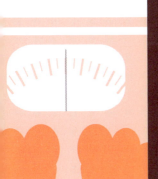

In addition, excess body fat increases inflammation throughout the body, including in your joints. Inflammation not only makes joints more tender, stiff, and sore, but it may actually cause osteoarthritis to progress faster. Inflammatory substances circulating in your body can also affect muscle function and sensitize nerves, leading to increased pain. Researchers at the Wake Forest University School of Medicine found that obese adults over the age of sixty with knee osteoarthritis who lost as little as 5 percent of their body weight noticeably decreased inflammation throughout their bodies.

Adopting an anti-inflammatory eating pattern such as the Mediterranean diet can help you slim down while also calming inflammation and tenderness in sore joints. However, losing weight can also cause bone mineral loss, weakening your bones and increasing your risk of fracture. Studies show that increasing your calcium intake while you're dropping pounds can help offset the loss of bone mineral, and adding a little more protein to the mix may further increase bone benefits, according to a 2008 study in the *Journal of Nutrition*. Plus, protein helps you hold on to metabolism-boosting muscle during weight loss.

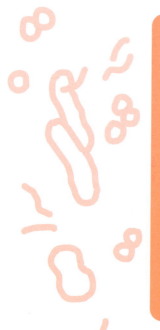

FEED YOUR GUT FERMENTED FOODS

Researchers in a study published in the medical journal *Aging Clinical and Experimental Research* in 2024 concluded that fermented dairy products significantly contribute to the beneficial effects of the Mediterranean diet. Fermented (lactic acid added to milk) foods include dairy products such as plain yogurt, buttermilk, and kefir. Kimchi, miso, and sauerkraut are also beneficial. Not only do fermented foods contain nutrients like calcium, they also have probiotics or "good bacteria," which improve gut health. The healthier your gut biome, the healthier your bones will be. That's because probiotics improve the absorption of calcium, regulate the metabolism of vitamin D, and improve immune function. Many fermented foods also contain prebiotics like inulin, which can be food for healthy gut bacteria to feed on. All good reasons to add fermented foods to your plate.

> **RECOMMENDED DAILY ALLOWANCE OF CALCIUM**
>
> A 2005 study in the journal *Sports Medicine* found that after a woman goes through menopause, exercise's ability to boost bone mineral density largely depends on adequate availability of dietary calcium. To be sure you're getting enough, follow the guidelines established by NIH:
>
> **Under fifty:** RDA is 1,000 mg of calcium per day
>
> **Over fifty:** RDA for men is 1,000 mg. RDA for women is 1,200 mg per day in divided doses.
>
> **Seventy and up:** Men and women need 1,200 mg per day in divided doses.

HABIT #2
Boost Bone Building Beyond Calcium and Vitamin D

Drinking milk is the only way to build strong bones.

FALSE

Although dairy products offer significant amounts of calcium and are frequently fortified with vitamin D, your bones may be better off if you get a good portion of these nutrients from both dairy and nondairy sources.

A study in the *American Journal of Clinical Nutrition* in 2023 examined the association between dairy products and the risk of fractures. This was a follow-up to the Health Study that involved 103,003 women with an average age of forty-eight from 1980 to 2004. It showed that two servings a day or more of total dairy (not counting yogurt) meant a lower risk of fracture.

But a meta-analysis and systematic review of research on this connection published in *Critical Reviews in Food Science and Nutrition* in 2020 showed no association between dairy consumption and a lower risk of fractures from osteoporosis. A 2009 review of studies in the *American Journal of Clinical Nutrition* noted that countries with the highest rates of dairy consumption also boast the highest rates of fracture from osteoporosis.

Given conflicting study results, filling your plate with a wide range of dairy and nondairy sources of calcium gives you the best bone benefit—good news for people who are lactose intolerant or who avoid dairy for other reasons.

Fruits and Veggies Benefit Bones

Calcium may be the most critical component of a bone-healthy diet, but vitamin D, potassium, magnesium, and other nutrients play indispensable roles as well. Studies show that eating more fruits and vegetables as part of a healthy eating plan, as in the Mediterranean diet and Dietary Approaches to Stop Hypertension (DASH) diet, can benefit your bones. A 2003 study in the *Journal of Nutrition*, for example, found that following the DASH diet for thirty days significantly reduced markers of bone turnover, which translates to less bone loss and lowered fracture risk. Add these bone builders to your diet to protect your frame as you get older. The Framingham Osteoporosis Study, which began in 1988 and 1989 as an offshoot of the Framingham Heart Study, found that upping fruit and vegetable intake improves bone mineral density.

Vegetables, fish, and fortified foods offer nondairy alternatives to help you reach the recommended amounts:

Vegetables in the kale family, such as broccoli, bok choy, cabbage, and mustard, spinach, and turnip greens, offer calcium that is as well absorbed as that in dairy products. For example, 1 cup (70 g) of cooked broccoli provides nearly 70 milligrams.

Nondairy sources of calcium include dried figs, white beans, almonds, tahini, and edamame (fresh soybeans). Studies are mixed, but soy seems to increase bone density and prevent fractures after menopause, when the most dramatic bone loss occurs.

Canned sardines and salmon, with their tiny edible bones, also supply calcium. In fact, a 3-ounce (85 g) serving of sardines contains more calcium (324 milligrams) than an 8-ounce (235 g) glass of nonfat milk (302 milligrams)! Fortified orange juice, soy foods, and breakfast cereals also contain good amounts, and some may offer bone-building vitamin D as well.

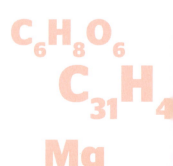

ESSENTIAL NUTRIENTS THAT BENEFIT BONES

Good bone health goes beyond calcium and vitamin D. Be sure to include all of these vitamins and minerals, whether from food or supplements:

Calcium. The USDA's 2024 Dietary Guidelines for Americans recommends that adults get three servings of dairy or calcium-rich foods every day. Fortified foods like cereal, orange juice, soy milk, and tofu are also good sources. If you take a supplement to make up the difference look for products marked "calcium carbonate" or "calcium citrate."

—

Vitamin D optimizes calcium absorption. Your body can make it when you expose your skin to sunlight. Or take a supplement of 400 IU per day if you're fifty to seventy, and 600 IU per day for those over age seventy. Fortified milk is the most common source of dietary vitamin D. Check the nutrition label for the vitamin D content of foods like cheese and yogurts.

—

Potassium helps your bones conserve calcium, possibly by preserving the body's acid/alkaline balance. Fruits and vegetables provide plenty of potassium, which researchers believe may be one of the main factors behind produce's bone benefits.

—

Magnesium increases calcium absorption and influences growth of crystals of hydroxyapatite, the mineral compound found in bone. Population studies have linked low magnesium intake to osteoporosis, and many people don't get enough. Find it in green leafy vegetables, whole grains, nuts, and dairy products.

—

Vitamin C "is essential for collagen formation and normal bone development," wrote Tufts University researchers in a 2008 study in the *Journal of Nutrition*. Bones are one-third collagen, which gives them their flexibility. Fruits and vegetables are your best sources for C and other antioxidants, including carotenoids such as beta-carotene and lycopene that protect against bone loss.

—

Vitamin K2 increases bone density and reduces fracture risk. Dark leafy greens, cruciferous vegetables, onions, and parsley contain vitamin K1, which your body can partly convert into beneficial K2 through digestion. Egg yolks, fermented dairy (such as cheese and yogurt), and fermented soy (such as miso and tempeh) are some of the few food sources of vitamin K2. Besides eating foods rich in K1 and K2, people with osteoporosis or osteopenia may want to supplement with 50 to 100 micrograms of K2 daily, and people with normal bone density may want to take 25 micrograms of K2. If you take anticoagulant drugs, check with your doctor before increasing vitamin K intake.

Dine on Vitamin D-Rich Foods to Delay Bone Breakdown

Vitamin D is critical for calcium absorption, and science is beginning to discover its importance in other body systems as well. If you don't get enough, your body secretes too much parathyroid hormone, which speeds up bone breakdown. In fact, some studies show that increasing calcium intake alone is not sufficient to protect you from fractures as you get older: Vitamin D makes the difference.

However, recent evidence indicates that a surprising number of people are deficient. Although your body can make vitamin D3 (cholecalciferol) from the UVB rays in direct sunlight, it's an unreliable source, and even some people who live in sun-soaked climates still don't make enough (not to mention rising concern about skin cancer risk). Plus, as you get older, your body is less efficient at producing vitamin D from the sun. Few foods contain vitamin D, but salmon, mackerel, tuna, sardines, egg yolks, and fortified cereals are good sources. U.S. dietary recommendations are 400 IU of vitamin D per day for adults age fifty to seventy, and 600 IU per day in those over age seventy.

In a 2008 study, Swiss researchers even suggested that all postmenopausal women and everyone over the age of sixty get 800 IU of vitamin D because it plays such a crucial role for bones and other aspects of health. Other experts recommend that people who get very little sun exposure take as much as 1,000 IU per day. Vitamin D is safe up to 2,000 IU, according to the Institute of Medicine.

To get that much, you'll almost certainly need to supplement in addition to eating these foods. Your multivitamin might contain some, and many calcium supplements now come with vitamin D as well. Look for D3 (cholecalciferol) on labels, since your body absorbs it better.

MAKE IT A HABIT: CALCIUM, VITAMIN D, AND MORE

Some vegetables, such as spinach, contain calcium, but also contain other nutrients that inhibit absorption of calcium. Other vegetables, such as kale, broccoli, bok choy, and cabbage, are calcium powerhouses. Add fermented dairy products like plain yogurt and kefir along with miso and sauerkraut to your plate for calcium, better gut health, and stronger bones. Vitamin D is necessary for calcium absorption. Foods such as salmon, mackerel, tuna, sardines, egg yolks, and fortified cereals are excellent sources. You also need potassium, magnesium, vitamin C, and vitamin K2.

Better Bones Shopping List
Next time you're at the store, stock up on these bone builders.

Calcium:
Dairy and fortified foods like milk, cheese, yogurt (vitamin D too), cereal, orange juice, soy milk, and tofu • Vegetables in the kale family, such as broccoli, bok choy, cabbage, and mustard, spinach, and turnip greens

Nondairy sources of calcium include dried figs, white beans, almonds, tahini, and edamame (fresh soybeans) • Canned sardines and salmon, with their tiny edible bones

Magnesium:
Green leafy vegetables, whole grains, nuts, and dairy products

Vitamin K2:
Egg yolks, fermented dairy (such as cheese and yogurt), and fermented soy (such as miso and tempeh)

Gut health/bone health:
Fermented foods such as plain yogurt, buttermilk, kefir, kimchi, miso, and sauerkraut; all are good for gut health, too

Calcium, potassium, magnesium, vitamin C, and more:
Choose a variety of fruits and vegetables.

HABIT #3
Diet Don'ts for Healthy Bones and Joints for Life

It's not enough to eat a diet rich in vitamins and minerals like calcium and vitamin D; it's also important to avoid diet don'ts.

TRUE

To protect your frame for the long haul, you need to do more than just eat foods rich in calcium, vitamin D, potassium, and other bone-benefiting nutrients. You should also minimize your intake of a few foods that can actually harm bone and joint health by triggering inflammation or leaching calcium from bones and blocking its absorption.

Nix Processed Foods, Trans Fats, Sugar, and Sodium to Protect Your Bones

Avoid processed foods. They contain a variety of health-sapping substances, including trans fats, refined carbs and sugar, and sodium. Trans fats, processed carbohydrates, and sugar all increase inflammation in your body, worsening stiffness, pain, and range of motion, and destroying cartilage in your joints. Inflammation also appears to accelerate bone breakdown and age-related bone loss. Aim to eliminate trans fats entirely and swap processed carbs for whole grains whenever possible.

Limit sugar. It's been implicated in increased osteoporosis risk, since it negatively affects the balance of minerals such as calcium and phosphorus needed for healthy bones. Try to limit the amount of added sugars in your daily diet to less than 6 teaspoons (about 100 calories or 24 g) for women and no more than 9 teaspoons (about 150 calories or 36 g) for men. Naturally occurring sugars, such as those in fruit and dairy products, are okay.

Watch the salt shaker. Excess sodium causes you to excrete more calcium, decreasing the amount available to bones. Sodium can also cause fluid retention and swelling, increasing pressure on tender joints. Manufacturers use salt and other high-sodium substances to preserve food and enhance flavor and texture, and processed and prepared foods such as canned vegetables, soups, deli meat, and frozen foods account for a whopping 77 percent of the average American's daily sodium intake.

The USDA recommends limiting your sodium intake to 2,300 milligrams (1 teaspoon [6 g] of table salt) per day. By far, the easiest way to cut back is to reduce the amount of processed and prepared foods you consume.

> **MAKE IT A HABIT: DITCH BONE DESTROYERS**
>
> Sugar decreases bone strength and may contribute to osteoporosis. Consume a maximum of 6 to 9 teaspoons (24 to 36 g) of added sugars a day. Salt causes you to excrete calcium, leaving less available for bones. Avoid processed foods and limit your salt intake to 1 teaspoon (6 g) or 2,300 milligrams of sodium per day. Caffeine leaches calcium from bones and interferes with its absorption. A little is okay (300 milligrams or less per day), but if you consume a lot of it, eat plenty of calcium-rich foods at other times to offset the risks. Regular sodas contain sugar, caffeine, and phosphoric acid that destroy bone health (and diet options aren't much better). Drink water, milk, or tea instead.

Watch What You Drink to Age Well

Although research is mixed about whether caffeine increases osteoporosis risk, studies do show that caffeine can cause bone loss and may leach calcium from bones and interfere with calcium absorption. That's especially problematic for older adults, who need all the calcium they can get to preserve their bones.

A 2001 study in the *American Journal of Clinical Nutrition* found that women over the age of sixty-five with high caffeine intakes had significantly higher rates of bone loss of the spine than did those with low intakes. A moderate intake (less than 300 milligrams per day) appears to be fine, but when you do consume caffeine, eat calcium-rich foods at other times to ensure maximum absorption of the mineral.

Sweetened beverages are bad for bones and joints because of their sugar content, which can lower bone mass and strength and aggravate inflammation. A 2008 study in the *Journal of Critical Care* found that soda drinkers, in particular, had reduced blood calcium and increased calcium excretion, setting them up for osteoporosis. Sugary soda that also contains caffeine is double trouble. But don't think you can simply reach for diet caffeine-free soda instead—a 2006 study in the *American Journal of Clinical Nutrition* found that even drinking diet and caffeine-free sodas a few times a week led to lower bone density in older women. Soda also contains phosphoric acid, which interferes with calcium absorption and contributes to imbalances that lead to additional loss of calcium. Choose healthier sips such as water, milk, and tea.

In addition to its other health benefits, moderate alcohol intake appears to boost bone density. However, heavy drinking disrupts calcium balance in the bones, reducing bone mineral density and increasing risk of fracture. Alcohol can also aggravate some forms of arthritis, such as gout. Limit your intake to two drinks or less per day for men or one or less per day for women for the best bone and joint protection.

HABIT #4
Use Natural Remedies to Strengthen Joints

Natural remedies can be a helpful adjunct and are often safer than some conventional treatments and therapies for joint and bone health.
TRUE

Natural remedies can help alleviate joint stiffness and pain. And because they carry less risk of harmful side effects than traditional treatments like NSAIDs and cyclooxygenase-2 (COX-2) inhibitors, they're a good thing to add to your medicine cabinet.

Protect Cartilage with Glucosamine and Chondroitin

Glucosamine and chondroitin sulfate are natural substances found in cartilage, the cushion between your joints. Glucosamine provides the raw material the body needs to manufacture long chains of sugar molecules (called *glycosaminoglycans*) found in cartilage and joint fluid. Chondroitin is the most plentiful type of glycosaminoglycan; it protects cartilage and attracts fluid to the connective tissue, bringing nutrients with it and allowing joints to absorb shock effectively.

MAKE IT A HABIT:
TAKE NATURAL PAINKILLERS

Studies suggest that glucosamine sulfate and chondroitin sulfate can relieve pain and stiffness and may even slow the progression of OA. Split the doses and take the supplements with food to avoid nausea and boost absorption. Glucosamine and chondroitin may interact with diuretics and blood thinners. Avoid chondroitin supplements made from shark cartilage, since they may contain heavy metals; most glucosamine supplements are made from shellfish, so read the label if you have a shellfish allergy. SAM-e, while expensive, reduces OA joint pain, as well as the need for NSAIDs, which may have harmful side effects. Pycnogenol, a pine bark extract, fights free radicals and calms inflammation, reducing pain and stiffness. *Boswellia serrata*, an anti-inflammatory herb, may relieve pain and swelling even up to a month after you stop taking it.

What the Science Shows

A meta-analysis of studies in 2018 in the *Journal of Orthopedic Surgery and Research* concluded that glucosamine reduced stiffness and chondroitin helped to relieve pain and improve joint function. A 2002 study in the *Archives of Internal Medicine* followed a group of people with knee osteoarthritis (OA) and found that those who took 1,500 milligrams of glucosamine sulfate every day for three years slowed the progression of the disease and improved pain, function, and stiffness. And a 2007 review of studies in the journal *Drugs and Aging* suggests that chondroitin sulfate combined with glucosamine sulfate—as opposed to glucosamine hydrochloride—is more likely to help improve OA symptoms. They also found "compelling evidence" that glucosamine sulfate and chondroitin sulfate stabilize cartilage loss and slow joint degeneration.

Supplement to Ease Age-Related Joint Pain

Most people with osteoarthritis can safely take 1,500 milligrams of glucosamine and 1,200 milligrams of chondroitin daily, the amount used in studies. Bump up the dose to 2,000 milligrams of glucosamine and 1,600 milligrams of chondroitin if you weigh more than 200 pounds (90.7 kg). You may want to divide the doses and take them throughout the day with food to prevent nausea and increase absorption. Allow three months to notice an improvement (some experts even suggest six months).

Talk to your doctor before taking glucosamine and chondroitin, since they may interact with drugs like diuretics and blood thinners. You should avoid chondroitin supplements made from shark cartilage, since they could be contaminated with heavy metals. And if you have a shellfish allergy, read ingredients labels carefully, since most glucosamine supplements are made from shellfish.

Select supplements from well-known manufacturers to increase the likelihood that they contain the stated amount and are free from contamination. You can also check the subscription-only Consumer Lab website, which offers independent testing of popular supplements by a variety of manufacturers. Or look for the U.S. Pharmacopeia (USP) label on supplements, which means that the ingredients have been verified by a third party.

Supplement with SAM-e to Soothe Sore Joints

Short for S-adenosylmethionine, SAM-e occurs naturally in cells. Your body produces less of it as you get older, which caused researchers to wonder if supplementing could help conditions like OA and other joint pain. Scientists suspect that SAM-e relieves pain by calming inflammation, and it may help keep cell walls flexible and allow for better cell communication as well. SAM-e also spurs production of the antioxidant glutathione, quelling free radicals. Lab and animal studies have shown SAM-e can stimulate the production of cartilage, but more research is needed to see if it can do the same in humans.

Studies show SAM-e can reduce joint pain and stiffness seemingly as well as traditional pain relievers like NSAIDs and COX-2 inhibitors. For example, researchers at the University of California, Irvine, compared SAM-e (1,200 milligrams) with celecoxib (Celebrex, 200 milligrams) for sixteen weeks to see how they reduced pain associated with knee OA. The researchers found that after two months, both treatments improved pain and joint function equally, although SAM-e took longer to take effect.

It's expensive to take the full recommended dose of SAM-e, although many people find that after an initial period of high dosing, they can maintain the effects with a smaller amount. Start with 400 milligrams three times a day for two weeks, then decrease to 200 milligrams twice a day thereafter.

People taking SAM-e seem to tolerate it well and are less likely to report problems than people using NSAIDs, but SAM-e can have side effects at the high dose, such as mild digestive distress—though it doesn't damage your stomach like NSAIDs can. Choose enteric-coated products labeled "butanedisulfonate," which is the most stable form. Some research suggests SAM-e also has an antidepressant effect, so unless your doctor says it's okay, you shouldn't use it if you are taking antidepressant medications to avoid interactions.

Try Pycnogenol to Relieve Arthritis Pain

Pycnogenol, the patented name for a French maritime pine bark extract, helps OA by fighting free radicals (it contains potent antioxidant compounds called bioflavonoids) and calming inflammation. A 2017 study in the medical journal *BMC Complementary and Alternative Medicine* found a reduction in inflammation in participants with severe osteoarthritis.

A 2008 study in the journal *Phytotherapy Research* found that OA sufferers who took 100 milligrams of Pycnogenol daily for three months had significantly reduced pain and stiffness and better joint function, and could walk much farther on a treadmill test compared to those given a placebo.

What's more, Pycnogenol takers were able to cut back on other pain-relieving medications such as NSAIDs and COX-2 inhibitors by 58 percent (and had 63 percent fewer gastrointestinal side effects as a result!). In a similar study published later that year, patients with mild to moderate OA took 150 milligrams of Pycnogenol daily and also experienced pain relief significant enough to allow them to reduce NSAID use.

Pycnogenol seems to be safe and well tolerated, but talk to your doctor if you'd like to try it, since it also has cardiovascular effects and could reduce your need for hypertension drugs. It may affect your blood sugar levels as well. Take 50 milligrams two or three times daily with meals.

Herbal Help for Healthy Joints

A 2020 study in *BMC Complementary Medicine and Therapies* examined the effects of *Boswellia serrata* (frankincense), an anti-inflammatory herb and its extract, and concluded that both improve pain, stiffness, and joint function. Other studies indicate that extracts help calm inflammation and improve OA symptoms such as pain and swelling.

A 2007 study in the *Indian Journal of Pharmacology*, for example, compared Boswellia extract (1,000 milligrams daily, divided into three doses) with a COX-2 inhibitor and found that, while Boswellia didn't take effect as quickly, within two months both treatments had similar benefits on OA symptoms. People who took Boswellia continued to notice improvements for up to a month after stopping the treatment, whereas the COX-2 inhibitor's effects dwindled as soon as that group stopped taking the drug.

Research shows that Boswellia prevents cartilage degradation. But more and better-designed studies in humans are needed to gauge the herb's benefit. As a 2008 review of studies in the *British Medical Journal* noted, "The evidence for the effectiveness of *Boswellia serrata* extracts is encouraging but not compelling."

HABIT #5
Reduce Midlife Joint Pain with Alternative Therapies

Alternative therapies are just woo-woo approaches that have little effect on bone and joint health.

FALSE

Beyond exercising, staying at a healthy weight, eating well, and taking supplements, alternative medicine therapies have shown promise for improving joint pain and other osteoarthritis symptoms. Acupuncture, transcutaneous electrical nerve stimulation, and massage can be helpful add-ons to other treatments and may be effective enough to allow you to reduce or even eliminate pain medications. Ask your doctor if it's worth giving these therapies a shot; insurance may cover or subsidize them.

Consider Acupuncture to Reduce Age-Related Stiffness

Acupuncture is probably the best-studied alternative therapy for treating joint pain and OA. Originating in China, acupuncture developed as a technique for restoring the balance of energy, or *qi,* in the body. Practitioners insert thin needles in points of the body that correspond to painful areas; the resulting stimulation of nerves, muscles, and connective tissue releases your body's natural painkillers (endorphins), suppresses stress hormones such as cortisol, and boosts blood flow. Electro-acupuncture is a common variation that uses pairs of needles and mild, continuous electric pulses traveling between them to provide additional stimulation.

Studies on acupuncture show a small, short-term benefit for pain, but because of the difficulty of devising a placebo treatment, the actual effect has proved tricky to measure. Still, the results are promising. A 2018 study in *Medicines* followed participants over a six-week period and found improvement in knee pain and mobility. Acupuncture has very few side effects and is considered quite safe if your practitioner is certified and uses sterile needles in a clean environment. However, you'll have to continue treatment to keep seeing results.

Try Out TENS to Block Pain Signals

Similar to electro-acupuncture, transcutaneous electrical nerve stimulation (TENS) uses a small, battery-powered machine with electrodes you attach to your skin to send a low-voltage electrical current along nerve fibers. These electrical impulses stimulate the nerve endings near painful joints, potentially blocking pain signals to the brain and triggering a release of endorphins. After initial training on how to use the machine, you can do the therapy at home. It's generally considered safe.

Several small trials have indicated that TENS can help relieve pain due to knee OA. And based on a review of current research, the Osteoarthritis Research International group, a team of sixteen medical professionals from six different countries, includes TENS as one of its twelve recommended nondrug treatments (along with acupuncture) to manage hip and knee OA.

A 2008 study in the *American Journal of Physical Medicine and Rehabilitation* found that combining hot packs and TENS reduced pain and improved function in women with knee OA. The TENS treatment group also showed increased muscle strength and better exercise performance compared to those who received ultrasound therapy plus hot packs, hot packs alone, or no treatment. And in a 2008 study in the journal *Chinese Medicine*, knee OA sufferers reported less pain and improved joint function after treatment with TENS. Those researchers found similar improvement with acupuncture and suggested that combining TENS and acupuncture would provide even greater benefits.

Massage for Greater Range of Motion and Joint Strength

Massage is helpful in reducing pain and increasing joint range of motion and strength. It works by encouraging blood flow to joints and stimulating endorphin release, and it may diminish pain-worsening stress hormones like cortisol as well. Because there are at least eighty different kinds of massage, gathering conclusive evidence about its effects on joint pain has proved difficult.

However, a 2006 study in the *Archives of Internal Medicine* found that Swedish massage twice weekly for a month, then weekly for another month significantly improved knee pain, stiffness, and joint function in OA sufferers compared to those who didn't receive massage. With very little downside, and potential benefits beyond relieving OA symptoms (it feels so good!), health care practitioners frequently recommend massage to alleviate OA pain.

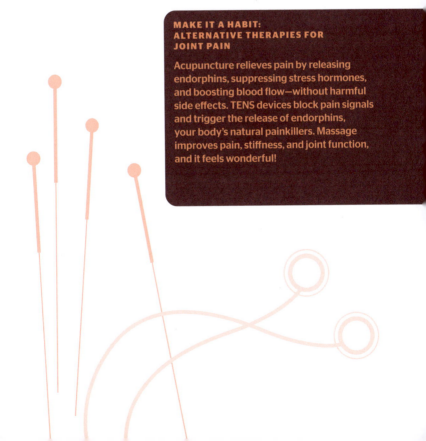

MAKE IT A HABIT: ALTERNATIVE THERAPIES FOR JOINT PAIN

Acupuncture relieves pain by releasing endorphins, suppressing stress hormones, and boosting blood flow—without harmful side effects. TENS devices block pain signals and trigger the release of endorphins, your body's natural painkillers. Massage improves pain, stiffness, and joint function, and it feels wonderful!

Powerful Habits to Turn Back the Clock on Your Heart

05

As we age, the heart gets a lot of attention from science and researchers. This means that it's an especially important area to keep an eye on.

Test your Heart IQ here >

TRUE

FALSE

(T) (F) *Exercise helps your heart, so plan to do it for thirty minutes at least twice a week.*

(T) (F) *Cholesterol levels and blood pressure rise with age, but natural remedies and lifestyle choices can make a big difference.*

(T) (F) *Focusing on a diet that has meat, dairy, and processed foods is beneficial for heart health.*

(T) (F) *Sudden, devastating events cause more cardiovascular stress than small daily stressors.*

(T) (F) *You need to get all your nutrition from food; supplements play no role in heart health.*

HABIT #1
Lower Your Cholesterol and Blood Pressure Naturally

Cholesterol levels and blood pressure rise with age, but natural remedies and lifestyle choices can make a big difference.
TRUE

Natural remedies and healthier lifestyle choices like diet and exercise can lower cholesterol, improve heart health, and lower blood pressure.

The Problem with Heart Disease

Your risk of cardiovascular disease increases as you get older, partly because cholesterol levels rise with age until you reach age sixty or sixty-five. Experts recommend keeping your total below 200 mg/dL; high levels (240 mg/dL and above) double your risk of heart disease. But total cholesterol doesn't tell the whole story. There are actually thirteen different kinds of cholesterol, including four types of low-density lipoproteins (LDL)—the "bad" cholesterol, and they each play a different role in cardiovascular health. A full lipid panel test reveals more about your risk of heart disease and the best way to keep cholesterol levels in check.

For high-density lipoproteins (HDL), the "good" kind that keeps cholesterol from building up in the walls of the arteries, the higher the numbers, the better. Less than 40 mg/dL is considered a major risk factor for heart disease, while 60 mg/dL and above actually protects against heart problems. Women often have higher HDL than men.

LDL accumulates in your arteries and creates fatty deposits called *plaques* that reduce blood flow. Rupturing of those plaques can cause serious heart and vascular problems. Ideally, your LDL should be less than 100 mg/dL (levels of 160 to 189 mg/dL are considered high), but women's LDL levels often rise with menopause.

Triglycerides are another type of blood fat that usually results from eating more calories than you burn (one reason why being overweight increases your risk of heart attack). High levels have been linked to coronary artery disease. You want your triglycerides to be less than 150 mg/dL.

If your cholesterol is high, you may not need to add another medicine to your regimen to get your levels back into a safe range. Talk to your doctor about trying these natural approaches before

> ## MAKE IT A HABIT: GO NATURAL TO IMPROVE HEART HEALTH AND BLOOD PRESSURE
>
> ### For Cholesterol:
>
> - *Reduce your intake of refined carbohydrates, such as white flour and sugar, and processed foods. Eat whole grains, legumes, fruits, and vegetables.*
>
> - *Exercise at a moderate pace for thirty to sixty minutes on most days of the week.*
>
> - *Switch to a margarine that includes plant stanols and sterols.*
>
> - *Supplement with artichoke extract, RYR, and fiber.*
>
> ### For Blood Pressure:
>
> - *Adopt the DASH diet, which emphasizes fruits, vegetables, whole grains, poultry, fish, and nuts, and limits fats, red meats, sweets, and sugary drinks.*
>
> - *Cut down on salt; flavor food with herbs instead.*
>
> - *Drink less alcohol (maximum of one drink a day for women, two drinks for men).*
>
> - *Get regular exercise and do strength training to lower blood pressure.*

taking a cholesterol-lowering drug that carries side effects. Give them about three months to show results. And even if you're already taking a cholesterol medication, adopting these habits can improve its effectiveness, potentially allowing you to reduce your dose.

Reduce your intake of refined carbs. As you get older, your weight tends to creep up. Excess weight lowers HDL while raising LDL and triglycerides, but losing as little as 5 to 10 pounds (2.3–4.6 kg) can help reverse that effect. One of the most effective dietary changes you can make is to reduce your intake of refined carbohydrates, such as white flour and sugar, and processed foods, which provide empty calories that get converted into triglycerides and extra pounds.

Eat more whole grains, legumes, fruits, and vegetables for their cholesterol-clearing fiber and plant stanols and sterols, which lower LDL. Swapping out saturated and trans fats for healthier monounsaturated fats—found in olive and canola oils, avocados, nuts, and seeds—and omega-3s is another smart step.

Regular exercise boosts HDL and lower triglycerides. Exercise can help you lose weight, thereby lowering LDL. A 2009 study in the *Journal of Physical Activity and Health* found that previously sedentary men who began exercising significantly improved measures of HDL, LDL, and triglycerides in just eight weeks. Aim for thirty to sixty minutes of moderate activity on most or all days of the week.

Red yeast rice. An eight-week study published in the 1999 *American Journal of Clinical Nutrition* showed that a proprietary Chinese red yeast rice (RYR) supplement reduced total and LDL cholesterol. Monacolin K, an ingredient in RYR, seems to be responsible for this beneficial effect. Look for a RYR supplement with the USP label to show the ingredients have been verified by a third party. Check with your health practitioner first, as the supplement can interact with alcohol, grapefruit, and certain medicines and herbal supplements like St. John's wort. In 2019, the authors of *The Methodist DeBakey Cardiovascular Journal* concluded that if cardiovascular risk factors are absent that the monacolin K in RYR is safe to take to manage mild to moderate cholesterol.

Artichoke leaf extract (*Cynara scolymus*) may reduce total cholesterol with few mild and quickly disappearing side effects, according to a 2009 review of studies. Preliminary research suggests it might also reduce LDL and triglyceride levels, but more studies are needed to confirm that effect. Take 1,800 to 1,920 milligrams a day, divided into two or three doses.

Take a fiber supplement like blond psyllium (found in seed husk and products) and oat bran also help lower total cholesterol and LDL, and ground flaxseed can help reduce triglycerides. For every 1 to 2 grams of soluble fiber you consume daily, you may lower your LDL by 1 percent, according to the Cleveland Clinic. Increase your fiber intake slowly to avoid digestive distress, but women should aim for 25 grams and men for at least 30 grams daily.

Adopt Habits to Control Blood Pressure without Drugs

High blood pressure or hypertension is one of the most common conditions among middle-aged and older adults. Blood pressure is the force of blood against the walls of arteries, and it's recorded as two numbers: systolic (as the heart beats) and diastolic (as the heart relaxes between beats). For the best heart health, your blood pressure should be below 120 systolic and 80 diastolic. A reading of 140/90 mm Hg or higher is considered high. There are no symptoms of high blood pressure, so check your blood pressure at least every two years. In the meantime, adopt these habits to regulate blood pressure and improve heart health:

Eat a heart-healthy diet to lower blood pressure. The DASH diet focuses on whole grains, poultry, fish, and nuts, and limits fats, red meats, sweets, and sugary drinks. Ease into this style of eating by serving two or more meatless meals per week, snacking on fruits and vegetables, and serving fruit for dessert.

Reduce sodium. Eating a lot of salt leads to your body holding excess fluid and increases the burden on your heart, wearing it out faster. Read labels to watch for sodium in prepared and processed foods such as canned vegetables, soups, deli meat, and frozen foods, and flavor food with herbs, not salt. Limit your sodium intake to 2,300 milligrams (1 teaspoon [6 g] of table salt) per day.

Limit alcohol, which can increase blood pressure, to one drink per day for women, or two for men. One drink is equal to 12 ounces (360 ml) of beer, 4 ounces (120 ml) of wine, 1.5 ounces (45 ml) of 80-proof distilled spirits, or 1 ounce (30 ml) of 100-proof spirits.

Get moving. In a 2006 review of studies, the researchers found that people with high blood pressure got the biggest benefit from exercise, reducing their systolic number by almost 7 points and their diastolic by nearly 5 points. As a bonus, exercise can also help you lose weight, reducing another risk factor for hypertension.

HABIT #2
Get the Nutrients You Need to Stave Off Heart Disease

Focusing on a diet that has meat, dairy, and processed foods is beneficial for heart health.
FALSE

Some of the healthiest foods for your heart are fruits and vegetables, nuts, and whole grains, according to a 2009 study in the *Archives of Internal Medicine*. These superstars offer key nutrients like antioxidants, B vitamins, and fiber, which help fight age-accelerating free radicals, improve heart and blood vessel function, and clear out artery-clogging cholesterol.

Amp Up Your Antioxidant Intake for a Stronger Heart

Plant foods are rich in free radical–fighting antioxidants called *flavonoids,* and diets that emphasize them are linked to lower death rates from cardiovascular disease, likely because the antioxidants improve the function of the endothelium, the smooth inner lining of the heart and blood vessels. Your endothelium stops working as well as you get older, and oxidative stress from free radicals speeds up that decline. Preliminary lab studies suggest that free radicals may also be responsible for dislodging plaques that have formed in blood vessels, potentially leading to a blockage and subsequent heart attack or stroke. And a 2009 study in the *Journal of Clinical Biochemistry and Nutrition* found that people with existing cardiovascular disease might be even more susceptible to the damaging effects of free radicals.

For heart health, vitamins C and E, carotenoids (such as beta-carotene and lycopene), and resveratrol are a few standout antioxidants. Vitamin E (found in wheat germ, nuts and seeds, and vegetable oils) prevents free radicals from attacking blood fats, and vitamin C (in citrus fruits, kiwi, and red and green peppers) relaxes blood vessels to boost blood flow while regenerating vitamin E.

Carotenoids (sources include carrots, cantaloupes, sweet potatoes, and spinach) may help prevent atherosclerosis, a buildup of plaque in blood vessels. And resveratrol, found in grapes and wine, acts directly as an antioxidant to relieve oxidative stress on the endothelium, but a 2009 study in the *Journal of Physiology and Pharmacology* found that it also boosts the performance of other important antioxidants in the body. Research clearly shows a heart benefit to boosting your intake of antioxidant-rich plant foods: Eat five to nine servings a day.

Bring on the B Vitamins to Reduce Stress and Inflammation

A 2010 study in the *American Journal of Clinical Nutrition* found that low vitamin B6 concentrations are connected to inflammation, increased oxidative stress, and metabolic conditions such as obesity and diabetes. Studies link low blood levels of folic acid with a higher risk of dying from heart disease and stroke. And B vitamins—particularly folic acid, B6, and B12—reduce levels of homocysteine, an amino acid linked to cardiovascular problems. Homocysteine increases with age, and it seems to accelerate atherosclerosis by damaging the inner lining of arteries and promoting blood clots.

Surprisingly, studies that have looked at supplementing with B vitamins to lower homocysteine levels show inconsistent results about their benefit to heart health. But experts agree on the importance of getting enough B vitamins in your diet to prevent heart problems and keep blood vessels young and healthy. The American Heart Association recommends getting 400 micrograms of folic acid a day. Citrus fruits, tomatoes, green leafy vegetables, and grain products are good sources, as are some fortified foods. You can find B6 in fortified cereals, beans, meat, poultry, fish, and some fruits and vegetables. Over the age of fifty, men need 1.7 milligrams daily, and women need 1.5 milligrams. Adults need 2.4 micrograms of vitamin B12 per day, but as you get older, you may not be able to absorb it as well; ask your doctor if this is a concern for you. Animal products, including fish, meat, poultry, eggs, and milk, are good sources of B12.

MAKE IT A HABIT: NUTRITION FOR HEART HEALTH

Eat five to nine servings a day of antioxidant-rich plant foods that are high in vitamins C and E, carotenoids, and resveratrol. Citrus fruits, tomatoes, green leafy vegetables, and grain products are good sources of folic acid; fortified cereals, beans, meat, poultry, fish, and some fruits and vegetables contain vitamin B6. Animal products such as fish, meat, poultry, eggs, and milk provide B12.

Fill up on soluble and insoluble fiber from whole grains, fruits, vegetables, and legumes. Limit sugar intake to 6 teaspoons (24 g) a day for women and 9 teaspoons (36 g) for men.

Feast on Fiber for Lifelong Benefits

The two types of dietary fiber, soluble and insoluble, each have benefits for your heart. Soluble fiber can lower LDL cholesterol, modestly lower blood pressure, and reduce heart disease risk. Insoluble fiber not only reduces the likelihood that you'll develop heart disease but also it can actually slow the progression of heart problems in high-risk people.

Eating high-fiber foods also makes you feel fuller, helping you keep your weight in check. Women should aim for 25 grams a day and men for at least 30 grams, but build up to that amount gradually to avoid stomach problems. Whole grains such as oats, barley, and brown rice are generally good sources of dietary fiber, as are beans, peas, carrots, cauliflower, apples, and nuts.

Dodge Diabetes as You Age by Decreasing Sneaky Sugars

Sugar is mainly empty calories, the opposite of heart-healthy nutrients. After you eat, your blood glucose (blood sugar) rises and your pancreas produces insulin to help muscle, fat, and liver cells use that blood glucose for energy. If your body does not make enough insulin or cannot use it well—insulin resistance—high levels of glucose build up in your blood, setting the stage for diabetes. If you have insulin resistance, are overweight, and have high blood pressure you may develop metabolic syndrome, which increases the risk of diabetes.

Type 2 diabetes is perhaps the most aging condition there is. Besides putting you at high risk for heart attack and stroke, having high blood sugar damages nearly every system in the body over time. Your doctor can use a fasting blood glucose test to check your blood sugar levels in the morning after eight hours of not eating. Normal blood sugar levels are 100 mg/dL or less.

Added sugars are the real problem because they typically break down very quickly and increase your blood sugar too fast. One of the most heart-healthy habits you can adopt is to decrease your sugar intake to help keep your blood sugar, insulin levels, and weight in check.

Limit to once-in-a-while treats. This includes soft drinks, cookies, cakes, ice cream, doughnuts, brown sugar on your oatmeal, and syrup on your pancakes.

Watch for sneaky sugars in your morning cereal, canned or frozen fruit, canned baked beans, spaghetti sauce, and other seemingly healthy foods.

Read the label. Look for names ending in "ose," such as maltose or sucrose, high-fructose corn syrup, molasses, cane sugar, corn sweetener, raw sugar, syrup, honey, or fruit juice concentrates.

Limit added sugars to no more than 100 calories per day, or about 6 teaspoons (24 g) of sugar, for women; for men, 150 calories or less per day, or about 9 teaspoons (36 g). That's a drastic cut from the typical American intake of 22 teaspoons (88 g) of sugar a day—about 355 calories!

HABIT #3
Tame Your Emotions (Anger, Depression, and Stress) to Take Years Off Your Ticker

Sudden, devastating events cause more cardiovascular stress than small daily stressors.
FALSE

Over time, the small daily stressors wear on us more than sudden, devastating events. Chronic stress ages your heart by increasing heart rate, blood pressure, and blood sugar and continually flooding your body with cortisol. High cortisol levels are linked to atherosclerosis, the buildup of plaque in the arteries, according to a 2008 study in the *Journal of Clinical Endocrinology and Metabolism*. In addition to the ways stress directly harms your heart, it can also tempt you to try other risky behaviors, such as smoking, drinking, overeating, or using drugs to relieve pressure.

How to Deal with Anger

Anger is a common response to stress, and evidence shows it can spike your heart rate and blood pressure, potentially raising your risk of heart problems. A 2009 study in the *British Journal of Health Psychology* demonstrated that suppressing anger has immediate and delayed cardiovascular consequences. In addition, a 2010 study in the *American Heart Journal* found that men and women who blamed others for their anger increased their heart disease risk as much as 31 percent. Men in the study who discussed their anger to resolve a situation, on the other hand, lowered their chances of developing heart disease. Make it a habit to deal with anger in a healthy way:

- **Choose your battles** *and resolve to fight fair. Don't be nasty, sarcastic, domineering, or hit below the belt, and avoid body language such as rolling your eyes.*

- **Don't suppress your anger** *and stew about it. That's a recipe for heart disaster.*

- **Find a trusted confidant.** *A friend you can vent to will help you move past the anger instead of dwelling on it.*

NOTES

> **MAKE IT A HABIT: STRESS BUSTERS**
>
> If you're angry, discuss it; don't let it stew. Be direct without being mean. Know your limits: Reduce the time you spend with people who push your buttons, and don't overschedule yourself.
>
> Practice gratitude, look on the bright side, get plenty of sleep, and pursue your hobbies to relieve stress.
>
> Volunteer to reduce isolation and depression, stay active, make friendships, and foster community.

Volunteer to Connect and Fight Depression

Volunteering offers a multitude of health benefits. It combats depression, fosters friendships, helps your community, and keeps you active. You can reap the health benefits by volunteering just two hours a week, or about 100 hours a year.

A 2009 study in the journal *Age and Ageing* found that older adults who volunteered or continued working past retirement age had fewer depressive symptoms, better mental well-being, and greater life satisfaction than those who retired without volunteering. And a 2010 study in the *Journal of Aging and Health* found that volunteering actually helps lift depression in people over sixty-five years old.

Volunteering helps combat depression by giving you a sense of purpose and connection, which is especially valuable if you don't currently get that from a job. Being socially active has a cyclical benefit too—if you connect with others, it can reduce depression, which in turn makes you more likely to stay socially engaged. Volunteering also keeps you physically active, which can reduce anxiety, besides keeping you fit and giving you more energy. Find a service opportunity at **www.VolunteerMatch.org,** or if there's a specific place you'd like to volunteer, ask at the front desk how you can get involved.

Reduce Stress to Live Longer, Happier

Stress is a fact of life, but you can learn to minimize certain triggers. For example, if long lines at the grocery store stress you out, try shopping at a less busy time. Stressed out by traffic? Try another route. It's also important to be realistic about what you can and can't fit into your schedule—and learn to say "no" to avoid overcommitting yourself. Same goes for that mile-long to-do list; prioritize your tasks to ensure the most important things get done.

Change Your Response to Stress for Long-Lasting Benefits
Exercise changes your body's reaction to stress by keeping your stress hormones balanced and boosting your mood. That can make all kinds of pressure-filled situations easier to bear. Getting enough sleep can help you handle stress better as well. Also, give yourself time to decompress daily by doing things you enjoy, whether it's pursuing a hobby, listening to music, or playing games with friends or loved ones. Even setting aside five minutes in the morning and in the evening to take a few slow, deep breaths can help.

Practice Gratitude, Reframe Negative Thoughts, Laugh
Cultivating happiness, or an optimistic outlook, helps tame tension, and research shows it can benefit your heart as well. A good way to do this is to focus on small things each day that you can be grateful for. Another is to reframe negative thoughts into reality-based positive ones. Laughter is another powerful stress buster, and research shows it can buffer stress's effects on blood pressure and help the inner lining of your blood vessels stay flexible and function better.

HABIT #4
Keep Your Heart Young and Strong with These Supplements

You need to get all your nutrition from food; supplements play no role in heart health.
FALSE

Solid science suggests a few supplements are good for overall heart health. If you're at high risk for heart disease, or if you already have cardiovascular problems, ask your health care practitioner if you could benefit from taking these supplements.

Omega-3's Antiaging Benefits

The omega-3 fatty acids EPA and DHA are found in oily fish such as salmon, mackerel, herring, lake trout, sardines, and albacore tuna, and study after study continues to extol their antiaging effects. A 2024 review of studies in *eClinicalMedicine*, part of The Lancet Discovery Science, involved over 149,051 participants and showed that omega-3 fatty acids improved a variety of cardiovascular outcomes.

A 2009 review of studies in the *American Journal of Therapeutics* noted that omega-3s can lower triglyceride levels, slow plaque buildup in your arteries (atherosclerosis), modestly lower your blood

MANAGE THE AGING SIDE EFFECTS OF HEART MEDS

If you do need to take prescription medicines, although most are safe and well tolerated, for some they can have troublesome side effects. Try these habits to feel better.

Stop statins' heart-aging side effects. These popular cholesterol-lowering drugs can cause headaches, digestive distress, and muscle and joint pain. They can also block the body's production of the antioxidant CoQ10, which is necessary for heart health, including fighting free radicals that accelerate cardiovascular aging, helping heart cells use oxygen efficiently, and keeping blood vessels young, flexible, and healthy. A heart-healthy diet and regular exercise can help you lower your dose and risk of side effects.

__ Avoid the drawbacks of blood pressure meds. Diuretics (such as hydrochlorothiazide), can deplete the body of potassium, magnesium, zinc, B vitamins, and CoQ10. Beta-blockers can cause depression, insomnia, cold extremities, fatigue, a slow heartbeat, and aggravated asthma symptoms. If you're taking diuretics, restore depleted nutrients by eating potassium-rich foods such as bananas and legumes, and take 600 milligrams of magnesium, 25 to 50 milligrams of zinc, and 60 to 90 milligrams of CoQ10 daily. If you're on beta-blockers, talk to your doctor about adjusting your dose or switching to another drug. And if you're taking any antihypertensive, eat a low-sugar, heart-healthy diet and exercise regularly to prevent diabetes.

__ Minimize the downside of antidiabetes drugs. Diabetes dramatically increases your risk of heart problems, so medications to control blood sugar, such as biguanides (Metformin), are an important part of treatment. But these drugs have the sneaky side effect of reducing levels of vitamins B6, B12, and folic acid. B vitamins support your nervous system, adrenal function, and metabolism. And shortages increase homocysteine levels, which raises your risk of kidney and heart disease, and possibly Alzheimer's. Take a daily multivitamin that contains B vitamins or a B-50 complex supplement with 400 micrograms of folic acid. Talk to your doctor about whether lifestyle changes can allow you to reduce your dose, or if you should switch to a different drug.

pressure, and protect against abnormal heartbeats and heart attack. If you don't get your omega-3s through food, you can supplement with fish oil capsules. To avoid possible contamination with dioxins, industrial chemicals called PCBs, and heavy metals like mercury, choose a reputable brand.

The American Heart Association recommends that most people get 500 milligrams of EPA and DHA per day for heart health (whether from fish or fish oil capsules). If you have coronary artery disease, take 1 gram per day, and those with high triglycerides should take 2 to 4 grams per day, divided into three doses. Check with your doctor before supplementing. If you're vegetarian, choose a supplement with DHA from algae, or take up to 3 grams of flax oil (your body can convert some of its alpha linolenic acid to omega-3s). Fish oil breaks down when exposed to light and heat, so look for a brand with natural preservatives like vitamin E or rosemary, purchase supplements from a store with high turnover, and store them in the refrigerator or freezer. To reduce fishy aftertaste and burps, take the capsules at the beginning of a meal and swallow them frozen.

Make Taking CoQ10 a Habit to Keep Your Heart Young

CoQ10 is a fat-soluble, vitamin-like substance found in every human cell. Responsible for producing energy, it also acts as an antioxidant and can benefit your brain as well as your heart. CoQ10 is naturally present in a variety of foods, including beef, soybean oil, sardines, mackerel, and peanuts, but people at risk for cardiovascular disease will likely need to supplement to get enough to see its heart-protective effects.

Studies show that CoQ10 benefits the heart by maintaining healthy blood vessels, preventing plaque buildup, and reducing the risk of plaque rupture. It also supports heart cells' high energy requirements and protects LDL ("bad") cholesterol from a process called oxidation that makes it harmful to blood vessels. A 2009 review of studies suggested that CoQ10 might help lower blood pressure as well.

Anyone who is taking statins, who has a family history of heart problems, or who is otherwise at risk for cardiovascular disease may benefit from supplementing. Take 50 to 150 milligrams per day in soft gel capsule form, and for best absorption, take it with a meal containing fat.

MAKE IT A HABIT: TAKE SUPPLEMENTS TO HEART

Eat oily fish (salmon, trout, mackerel, sardines, and tuna) to get the heart-healthy benefits of omega-3s. If you don't eat enough fish, supplement with fish oil capsules, preferably frozen and with a meal to reduce fishy aftertaste and burps. Take CoQ10 to increase energy and fight heart-aging free radicals. CoQ10 also benefits the heart by reducing plaque buildup and the risk of plaque rupture.

Powerful Habits to Turn Back the Clock on Your Immune System

06

Immunity is like being inside a protective bubble. It keeps us from getting sick and helps us recover faster. As we age, it's important to reinvigorate our immunity to make sure that it's robust so it's there when we need it.

What's your Immunity IQ?

TRUE

FALSE

(T) (F) **All stress is bad, when it comes to your immune system.**

(T) (F) **When you don't get enough sleep or have poor sleep quality, it impacts immunity.**

(T) (F) **Cultivating a positive mindset helps improve how your immune system functions.**

(T) (F) **Free radicals have little to no impact on your immune system.**

(T) (F) **Herbal remedies like ginseng, echinacea, and astragalus can help boost immunity.**

(T) (F) **Getting a cold, sinus infection, or strep throat doesn't factor into more serious illnesses like the flu and chronic diseases.**

HABIT #1
Use Mind-Body Therapies to Stop Aging Stress

All stress is bad, when it comes to your immune system.
FALSE

Short-term stress can actually boost your immune system, sending it into overdrive to protect you from infection and disease. But chronically elevated levels of stress hormones, like cortisol and adrenaline, put you in a constantly heightened state of arousal. Inflammation damages your body over time and makes your immune system less able to respond to signals to turn off that inflammation.

Help the Thymus Gland by Learning to Handle Stress Better

Aging affects your immune system in several ways. By the time you reach sixty, your thymus gland has mostly stopped producing T cells, which are critical to immunity. That means your body has to depend on the T cells you've already stored up, and as those cells gradually change and die off, you're less able to make antibodies and your immune system doesn't "remember" past illnesses as well. That "memory" is why you normally don't get infected with the same strain of a cold virus a second time.

Additionally, a 2008 study in the journal *Neuroimmunomodulation* found that as you get older, your immune cells—especially white blood cells—are fighting off more inflammatory compounds and free radicals with fewer antioxidant defenses to draw from. By itself, that's enough to raise your risk of infection (such as flu and pneumonia), cancer, and autoimmune diseases as you age. But chronic stress adds an extra burden, suppressing your immune system and wearing it down even faster.

Make These Practices a Habit to Boost Your Immunity

To keep your immune system strong and healthy as you get older, managing chronic stress is crucial. You may not be able to change the source of your stress, but by taking time for yourself you can change your response to anxiety-inducing situations. Try these proven stress busters to start.

Pursue hobbies. People who participate in a variety of fun activities in their leisure time have reduced cortisol levels, along with several other indicators of good health, according to a 2009 study in *Psychosomatic Medicine.*

Be mindful. A mindfulness-based stress reduction program of twenty minutes of meditative breathing and stretching per day was enough to lower workers' stress levels by nearly 10 percent, according to a 2009 study in the journal *Health Education and Behavior*. And moderate exercise boosts immunity as well.

Try aromatherapy. Surround yourself with calming scents to strengthen your immune system. Study participants who sniffed lavender or rosemary essential oils for five minutes lowered cortisol levels and increased their bodies' abilities to fight off aging free radicals, according to a 2007 study in the journal *Psychiatry Research*. If you can, bring in a few sprigs of fresh lavender or a potted rosemary plant—exposing yourself to nature even in small doses can snuff out stress.

LISTEN TO MUSIC TO BOOST IMMUNE FUNCTION

As you get older, your immune system grows less responsive and doesn't communicate as well with your nervous system. That means, for example, that your white blood cells can't read signals from your nervous system to turn off inflammation. Music helps to reestablish that communication and bring hormone and neurotransmitter levels back into balance. Both listening to and making music in a choir or a band (communal experiences also offer mental, social, and physical stimulation that boost brainpower) or on your own boosts your mood, makes you more resilient to stress, and enhances memory and focus. Choose relaxing music with a slow tempo you enjoy or faster songs when you're exercising to destress for an energy boost.

Connect with nature. Japanese researchers found that volunteers who stayed in a hospital room decorated with natural materials had 20 percent lower cortisol levels than those who stayed in a typical hospital room. Going for a walk in the woods (green forest bathing) can help to reduce stress. Go to the beach to benefit from negative ions caused by crashing water to boost your mood.

Do yoga. Poses and stretches like Tree, Downward Dog, Extended Triangle, Cat/Cow, and Child's Pose release tension and help you relax. Yoga also makes you more flexible, improves balance, and centers you in the present moment, which also reduces stress.

Laugh often. Not only does it make you feel good, but it boosts your immune system as well, and researchers believe that the benefit stems from stress reduction. In a study published in *Alternative Therapies in Health and Medicine*, researchers asked fifty-two healthy men to watch a comedy video. After that one hour of laughing, several markers of immune function increased for up to twelve hours afterward. The act of laughing can increase the activity and number of natural killer cells in the immune system.

Use the Power of Touch for Lifelong Immunity

Your hardworking immune system naturally slows down as you get older, leaving it less responsive and able to protect you from infection and disease. But these therapies and habits can help:

Massage improves several markers of immune function, such as lymphocyte, T cell, and natural killer cell counts. Massage reduces stress and the release of the stress hormone cortisol, which destroys natural killer cells—the immune system's front line of defense—and lowers immune-suppressing cortisol levels. Massage also increases the production of feel-good neurotransmitters dopamine and serotonin, helping prevent or lift depression, which increases cellular immunity. Self-massage, such as a foot rubdown or hand massage, also reduces stress and anxiety and boosts mood.

Touch. Handshakes, hugs, holding hands, back rubs, snuggling, and massage increases the production of oxytocin, a hormone made in the brain that stimulates our desire to connect with others. It can increase feelings of trust, generosity, and love, and studies show it also lowers cortisol levels and several markers of inflammation, potentially helping a declining immune system keep inflammation levels in check.

Sex reduces stress and helps you sleep better. A 2004 study in the journal *Psychological Reports* found that men and women who had sex once or twice a week had higher levels of an immune system protein called *immunoglobulin A (IgA)* than those who had less sex. Your body also produces sky-high levels of oxytocin during orgasm (self-love counts), which bolsters your immunity.

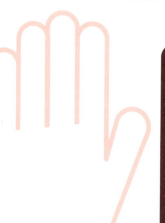

> **MAKE IT A HABIT: STRESS BUSTERS**
>
> Pursue hobbies, practice mindfulness, try aromatherapy, and get out in nature to get "me" time and destress.
>
> Do yoga, exercise, stretch, or breathe deeply for at least twenty minutes a day to lower your stress levels by 10 percent.
>
> Laugh more. Watch comedies, hang out with funny friends, or read humor on a regular basis to improve immunity.
>
> Use touch to reduce stress, improve mood, and bolster the immune response.
>
> Listen to or make music to reduce stress and improve immunity.

HABIT #2
Don't Skimp on Sleep as You Get Older

When you don't get enough sleep or have poor sleep quality, it impacts immunity.
TRUE

While you're sleeping, your body is busy repairing itself. When you don't get enough sleep, or don't sleep deeply, that healing doesn't happen as well. That can spell big trouble for your immune system as you get older, putting you at increased risk of infection and disease.
In a healthy brain, substances related to immunity interact with neurochemical systems to regulate your sleep. But as you age, communication between your immune system and your nervous system begins to break down. A lack of sleep can further upset the balance, aging your immune system so it can't protect you as well.

Sleep = Immunity

In a 2021 study in *Nature*, researchers surmised that sleep does support immune function and helps us be more resilient when it comes to preventing infection and inflammation. Although they don't know exactly how sleep impacts immunity, and more studies are needed, some suspect that your body's circadian rhythms affect immune system cells, or that sleep may reduce immunity-weakening oxidative stress (in effect, functioning as an antiaging free radical fighter). The sleep-regulating hormone melatonin, which also decreases with age, influences several aspects of immunity as well. In fact, researchers are currently investigating whether supplementing with melatonin can restore immune function in older people.

You need at least seven hours a night to reach healing rapid-eye movement (REM) sleep, evidence indicates. A 2009 study in the *Archives of Internal Medicine* found that volunteers who got less than seven hours of sleep nightly for two weeks were nearly three times as likely to develop a cold when exposed to a virus. Thankfully, putting the following sleep habits into practice may be enough to restore that nightly healing process and keep your immune system functioning at its best as you get older.

> **MAKE IT A HABIT: SLEEP SOUNDLY**
>
> Keep a journal to determine if your diet, exercise routines, anxiety over a personal issue, or other factors are at the root of your sleeping problems. Practice good sleep hygiene. Keep the bedroom dark and quiet, stick to a regular sleep/wake schedule, and, if needed, use a white noise machine to sleep well. Exercise regularly, but avoid working out and doing other stimulating activities before bedtime. Instead, soothe yourself by drinking warm tea or milk. If you still aren't sleeping well, try taking valerian or melatonin.

Smart Strategies to Help You Sleep Like a Baby

In later life, many people don't sleep as well as they used to, due to medications, hormonal shifts, changing responsibilities, and chronic conditions. For example, common drugs like beta-blockers for high blood pressure and NSAIDs for joint pain significantly lower melatonin production, thereby aggravating insomnia. If you have trouble sleeping, keeping a sleep journal in which you record activities, what you eat and drink, how you feel, or other factors that influence how well you sleep may shed some light on what's interfering with a good night's rest. If your sleep problems last longer than two weeks, talk to your doctor about possible underlying factors. Practice good sleep hygiene habits to set the stage:

- **Reserve your bed** (and bedroom) for sleeping and sex.

- **Avoiding stimulating activities and stimulants** like reading the news, using nicotine, and consuming caffeine before bed. Nix alcohol for several hours before bedtime. If you're sensitive, you may need to cut all of these substances out completely.

- **Stick to a regular sleep/wake schedule** even on weekends. Exercise regularly, but not in the few hours before you go to bed.

- **Tame anxiety.** Try putting your thoughts in a journal or make a to-do list so you don't keep ruminating.

- **Keep your bedroom dark and quiet** to minimize sleep interruptions and ensure you get enough immune-boosting REM sleep. Use a white noise machine to mask unwanted sounds.

- **Limit naps.** Napping to make up for lost sleep may actually make it harder to fall and stay asleep at night, when the immune system needs it most, so keep daytime snoozing to a minimum if possible.

Try Natural Remedies to Sleep Better

If you still have trouble falling asleep, have a few sips of chamomile tea or warm milk before bed. Both have relaxing properties, and having something warm in your stomach can be comforting. Two of the best natural sleep aids are valerian (*Valeriana officinalis*) and melatonin. Valerian, an herbal sedative that's been used for centuries, is non-toxic and not addictive, but some people find it leaves them feeling fuzzy-headed in the morning. If you'd like to try it, take one or two capsules of a product standardized to 1 percent valerenic acid thirty minutes before bedtime.

Supplemental melatonin is also available over the counter. Other than causing an increase in dreaming, it has no known side effects. Dr. Andrew Weil, M.D., an integrative physician, author, and professor, recommends taking 2.5 milligrams at bedtime occasionally if needed. He prefers sublingual tablets that dissolve when you place them under the tongue, but capsules are also an option. For regular use, a much lower dose (0.25 to 0.3 milligrams) may be effective.

DO AEROBIC EXERCISE THE RIGHT WAY TO MAINTAIN IMMUNITY

Along with eating well, aerobic exercise can boost your immune system in the short and long term, providing extra protection against infection and disease as your body's natural defenses begin to decline. A 2006 study in the *American Journal of Medicine* found that women who did forty-five minutes of moderate-intensity exercise five days per week for a year had increasingly improved immunity, to the point that by the end of the study they were three times less likely to catch a cold. Burning calories also helps you lose weight, which reduces immunity by aging the thymus system and slowing its production of T cells, a type of white blood cell.

Exercise helps you sleep better and be more likely to eat a healthy diet, both of which help keep your immune system young and strong. Thirty to forty-five minutes of moderate exercise on most days of the week will strengthen your immune defenses. Don't overdo it. High-intensity exercise dampens the immune response. If you do exercise for more than ninety minutes, consume carbs and supplement with quercetin or curcumin to counteract increased stress and restore white blood cell function.

HABIT #3
See the Glass as Half-Full to Bolster Immunity

Cultivating a positive mindset helps improve how your immune system functions.
TRUE

A positive outlook confers many health benefits, including lower blood pressure and better recovery from surgery. And research shows it can also improve immunity, both by mediating immune-suppressing stress and actively boosting several markers of a healthy immune system. For older adults, the difference may even be significant enough to offset the natural decline of their immune systems.

A generally sunny disposition, as well as having specific high hopes, seems to buffer the damaging effects of stress on the immune system. For instance, people characterized as being anxious, hostile, and depressed were three times more likely to get sick when exposed to a cold or flu virus than their happy, lively, and calm counterparts, noted a 2006 study in *Psychosomatic Medicine*.

Feeling like you have control over your circumstances makes a difference too. When study participants had actual or perceived control over a stressor, the optimists had better natural killer cell function than their pessimistic peers, reports a 2005 study in the journal *Brain, Behavior, and Immunity*.

Studies have shown that a positive mood is associated with stronger cellular immunity. On the flip side, a 2009 study in the journal *Brain, Behavior, and Immunity* found that pessimism actually accelerated aging and weakened immune function in postmenopausal women. Making an effort to be more positive may be a buffer against depression down the road, which can help you thrive in the face of adversity, says Dr. Mathers.

Depression, which is linked to feelings of hopelessness and pessimism, can be harmful to health. Depressed people generally don't exercise as much, sleep as well, or eat as healthfully—neglecting the building blocks of immunity. Depression also triggers inflammation and suppresses natural killer cell activity and the creation of T cells that fight off infection.

Cultivate Optimism for a Stronger Immune System

Evidence indicates that optimism can be learned. It is a choice as much as a perspective. So how do you become more positive if you don't naturally have an upbeat outlook? And since optimists do better than pessimists in almost every aspect of life—including immunity—experts agree it's worth making the effort. Try the four-step process of confronting negative thoughts that Dr. Mathers uses to help his patients feel more optimistic:

1 *Recognize negative thought patterns.*

2 *Label the thoughts as detrimental to your well-being.*

3 *Identify positive alternatives.*

4 *Make a concerted effort to replace the negative thoughts with the alternatives.*

Let Go of Grudges and Boost Optimism for a Younger Immune System

Did you know that forgiveness is critical to maintaining good health? First, it relieves stress, which suppresses your immune system, and second, forgiveness is essential for healthy relationships, and a strong social network acts as a further buffer to the harmful, age-accelerating effects of stress and depression. All of this helps you look on the bright side of life.

Keep in mind, deciding to forgive someone is not the same as emotionally forgiving someone, according to a 2007 study in the *Journal of Behavioral Medicine*. Decisional forgiveness, or controlling your behavior, might reduce outward hostility, but it doesn't switch off the stress response that ultimately wears down your immunity. So your grudge is still damaging you, not them.

MAKE IT A HABIT: CHOOSE OPTIMISM

Recognize that negative thought patterns are harmful to your health; identify positive alternatives and work to change your thinking. Be willing to let go of grudges that cause stress and suppress your immune system and can cause depression.

Surround yourself with optimistic people and friends who make you laugh. Avoid pessimists; their dour attitudes can be contagious. Practice gratitude for the small and big things in your life.

Emotional forgiveness—changing your thinking, emotion, and motivation (which ultimately leads to changed behavior)—has more direct health benefits because it helps you move from a place of negativity and stress to a more hopeful, positive attitude. And staying in that happier frame of mind bolsters your immune system.

Adopt a disposition of forgivingness, which means making it a habit to extend grace to yourself and others. Research shows that highly forgiving individuals showed less depression and stress and greater subjective and psychological well-being than their less forgiving peers, according to a 2006 study in the journal *Personality and Individual Differences*.

Forgiveness doesn't mean that you're saying what happened didn't matter, or that you're condoning bad behavior, either. Rather, you are refusing to let bitterness take hold and harm your health. In fact, middle-aged and older adults who showed higher levels of forgiveness toward others reported better physical and mental health, according to a 2001 study in the *Journal of Adult Development*. Forgiveness takes you out of the victim's role, puts you back in control, and frees your immune system to function at its best for a long, healthy life.

Surround Yourself with Positive People (and Avoid Negative People)

Surrounding yourself with cheerful people can also help you change your perspective. If you're having trouble breaking out of negative thought patterns, you might even ask a particularly positive friend how she might see your situation in a better light. Funny friends who can help you laugh, at yourself or your circumstances, are also worth seeking out. Laughter boosts your mood, making it easier for you to focus on positive thoughts, and it also relieves stress that can further weaken an aging immune system.

Pessimism is contagious, so minimize the time you spend with complainers, cynics, and other negative people. Talk to your doctor if you suspect you're depressed. And don't let pessimism make you passive: "An optimistic person takes hold of the possibility of a [positive] outcome and often works or even fights to make that happen," notes Mathers.

Practice Gratitude

Making it a habit to notice small things that you're grateful for like a sunny day, a good meal, or an entertaining TV show can help to boost your mood. Big things like your friends, your work, and your family, including your pets, are important as well when it comes to filling up your gratitude cup. Make it a practice to stop several times a day and notice what's good in your world. Over time, this will help you see things in a more positive light. Use the worksheet opposite to get started.

GRATITUDE HABIT TRACKER

Write down three or four things that you're grateful for. Repeat this practice to fill up your gratefulness cup and boost your mood. Create a gratitude journal to continue your practice and make it a habit.

I'm Grateful for...

I'm Grateful for...

I'm Grateful for...

I'm Grateful for...

I'm Grateful for...

I'm Grateful for...

HABIT #4
Supercharge Your Diet with Immune-Boosting Foods

Free radicals have little to no impact on your immune system.
FALSE

Free radicals accelerate aging throughout the body, and your immune system is no exception. In fact, research shows that your immune system, especially your white blood cells, faces increasing amounts of free radicals as you get older. Fighting off that oxidative damage with antioxidants, therefore, is a surefire strategy to keep your immune system young and strong.

Antioxidant vitamins, minerals, and nutrients protect and repair immune system cells, improving your body's ability to defend itself against colds, flus, and other infections. Research shows that several other foods offer protective compounds as well, and they all fit into a healthy diet—even antioxidant-rich dark chocolate! In general, your body absorbs nutrients better from foods than from supplements, so round out your diet with these superfoods and you'll be well on your way to super immunity.

GET YOUR VITAMIN D FROM FOOD, NOT THE SUN

Too much UV radiation can actually suppress your immune system. Two kinds of UV wavelengths reach the earth: UVA and UVB. UVB rays increase your risk of DNA changes that can develop into skin cancer, and UVA rays create free radicals that not only damage DNA but also impair your immune system.

— Exposure to these immune-suppressing UVA rays causes a defect in the development of T cells (a type of white blood cell) that impairs their ability to become "long-term memory" cells, which allow your immune system to remember and defend against illnesses and bugs you've already encountered, such as chicken pox. Since your body gradually stops producing naïve T cells by the time you reach your mid-sixties, you need memory T cells to keep you healthy.

— Sun exposure does allow skin to synthesize vitamin D, but you're better off getting vitamin D from foods and supplements, since as you age, your body becomes less efficient at producing vitamin D from the sun, and because the risks of sun exposure to your skin and your immune system are so high.

Slow Aging with Antioxidant-Rich Fruits and Vegetables

An abundance of antioxidants such as the B vitamins, vitamins C and E, beta-carotene, and flavonoids make fruits and vegetables immune-strengthening powerhouses. Aim for five to nine servings per day and eat a variety of brightly colored produce to ensure you get a good mix of all the antiaging antioxidants they offer.

For example, bright orange-hued sweet potatoes and carrots contain vitamin C and beta-carotene, bright blue and red berries boast anthocyanins and other flavonoids, and bright red watermelon provides the powerful antioxidant glutathione. For the best free radical–scavenging benefits, eat these foods raw or lightly steamed. Overcooking can destroy the antioxidants, and boiling leaches nutrients into the cooking water.

> **MAKE IT A HABIT: FOODS AND EXERCISE FOR SUPER IMMUNITY**
>
> Eat a rainbow of colorful fruits and vegetables to reap antiaging antioxidants. Mushrooms and garlic will help you fight off viral infections and other illnesses. Have a serving of nuts or a little red meat for minerals that boost immunity.
>
> Drink white, green, or black tea (caffeinated or decaf) for a dose of vitamin C and antioxidants. Practice aerobic exercise for thirty to forty-five minutes most days of the week to boost immune function. Avoid too much exposure to the sun because it can impair immune function.

Broccoli and other cruciferous vegetables such as cabbage contain glutathione and the antioxidant compound sulforaphane. When researchers treated older mice with sulforaphane, the compound increased their immune response to the level of younger mice, according to a 2008 study in the *Journal of Allergy and Clinical Immunology*.

Mushrooms offer a few particular benefits as well. Asian mushrooms (shiitake, maitake) contain beta-glucans, a type of carbohydrate that boosts the immune system. And regular button mushrooms provide antioxidants such as selenium, as well as the B vitamins riboflavin and niacin. Riboflavin increases resistance to bacterial infections, while niacin reduces oxidative stress and inflammation. Lab and animal studies also indicate mushrooms have antiviral, antibacterial, and antitumor effects.

Garlic gets its odor from the sulfur compound allicin, which also increases the production of white blood cells. In addition, a 2007 study in the *Journal of Interferon and Cytokine Research* found that eating 2 grams (less than a teaspoon) of fresh garlic stimulated the production of nitric oxide and interferon alpha, which activate immune cells and help fight viral infections. Fresh garlic seems to be best, but if you don't like the taste, peel, chop, and let it sit fifteen to twenty minutes before gently cooking to activate immune-boosting enzymes.

Eat a Daily Serving of Other Immune-Boosting Foods

White, green, and black tea are some of the healthiest drinks around, offering vitamin C and antioxidant flavonoids and polyphenols. (Caffeinated and decaf varieties work equally well.) Nuts also provide antioxidant vitamins and minerals. Almonds, for example, offer nearly 50 percent of the recommended daily amount of vitamin E per ¼ cup (36 g) serving. They also boast the B vitamins riboflavin and niacin. Brazil nuts provide exceptional amounts of selenium—one nut contains almost 100 micrograms, or nearly twice the recommended daily amount. A 2008 review of studies noted that selenium supports the immune system in several ways, partly by offsetting the effects of aging on immunity.

The Importance of Selenium and Zinc
Red meat also serves up selenium and the immune-boosting mineral zinc. Zinc speeds wound healing and may have an antiviral effect as well. Low levels of zinc impair immunity, decrease resistance to germs, and are linked to more frequent and severe bouts of pneumonia in older adults (and, as a result, longer rounds of treatment), noted a 2010 study in *Nutrition Reviews*. Oysters and wheat germ are also good sources.

Add Friendly Bacteria
Probiotics, or "good" bacteria, may spur your immune system to fight disease. They're especially beneficial if you've been taking antibiotics, which wipe out all bacteria—good and bad—in your system. That can compromise your immune response—specifically, the function of white blood cells called *neutrophils*, suggests a 2007 study in *Nature Medicine*. Yogurt with live and active cultures is a prime source, but more and more foods are being fortified with these friendly bacteria.

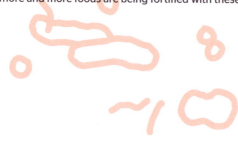

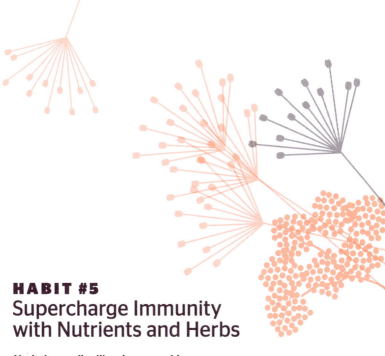

HABIT #5
Supercharge Immunity with Nutrients and Herbs

Herbal remedies like ginseng, echinacea, and astragalus can help boost immunity.
TRUE

In addition to getting enough rest, exercising regularly, and eating plenty of antioxidant-rich foods—the building blocks of healthy immunity—you may want to consider taking an herbal supplement to counteract the natural decline in your immune system as you get older. Read labels carefully and obey warnings, and let your doctor know you'd like to try them, since some herbs can interact with drugs or other natural remedies.

Prevent Immune System Decline with North American Ginseng

The antioxidant and anti-inflammatory herb North American ginseng (*Panax quinquefolius*) contains compounds called *ginsenosides* and *polysaccharides* that seem to be responsible for the herb's immune-boosting effects. It broadly supports the immune system and protects against stress, and you can take it indefinitely to help shore up your immune system as it naturally slows down with age.

A 2009 review of studies in *Evidence-Based Complementary and Alternative Medicine* concluded that while North American ginseng doesn't reliably reduce the incidence or severity of colds and respiratory infections, it appears to shorten their duration. The herb might also exert antitumor effects: A ginseng extract slowed the spread of and killed human colon cancer cells in lab tests, according to a 2010 study in *Phytomedicine*.

Preparations and quality of this herb vary widely, so look for standardized products that indicate the ginsenoside content and follow the package dosing directions. Take it regularly throughout the cold and flu season, or at the first sign of a cold to shorten its duration. If you use it long term, take two to three weeks off every four months. People with fibroids or with a history of breast cancer shouldn't take it, and it can interact with some drugs for heart disease, diabetes, and depression.

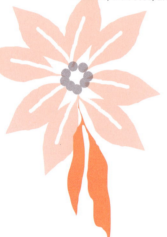

MAKE IT A HABIT: TAKE POWERFUL HERBS

Take North American ginseng indefinitely to boost immunity and shorten the duration of colds. Try astragalus, long used in China, to improve disease resistance and fight chronic infections. Take echinacea for up to ten days to shorten the duration of upper respiratory infections. Use elderberry extract to shorten colds and reduce symptoms.

Increase Your Immunity with Astragalus

Astragalus membranaceus is another nontoxic herb you can take indefinitely to improve disease resistance and help fight off chronic or recurrent infections. Despite its long history of use in China, it hasn't been studied often in humans. Astragalus reduced production of several inflammatory markers in mouse cells, according to a 2008 study in the *Journal of Medicinal Food*. In other lab and animal studies, astragalus increased T-cell counts in samples with low levels (common in older adults), enhanced antibody responses, and improved white blood cells' ability to eliminate harmful intruders.

Additionally, astragalus restored the white blood cell response of older mice to levels normally found in younger mice and partially reestablished immune function in mice with tumors or other immune problems, noted a 2007 study in the *Journal of Ethnopharmacology*. In one of the few human studies, patients with depressed immune systems due to stomach trauma were given astragalus, which helped restore cellular immunity. And in a pair of studies investigating astragalus, echinacea, and licorice, researchers found that each of the supplements boosted immune cell activity for up to seven days (the combination was even more powerful).

Look for standardized extracts of astragalus in liquid, capsule, or tablet form. Follow the daily dosing directions on the package. People who are on immune-suppressing drugs to treat cancer or who are organ-transplant recipients should not use astragalus.

Shorten the Duration of Colds with Echinacea

Also called purple coneflower, echinacea (*Echinacea purpurea* and *Echinacea angustifolia*) is one of the most-studied herbs for cold prevention. Lab and animal studies indicate it has antiviral and anti-inflammatory properties and activates white blood cells. And while studies in humans show echinacea doesn't prevent colds, it does seem to shorten their duration. A 2007 study in the *International Journal of Sports Medicine* noted that volunteers who took echinacea for four weeks had higher levels of antibodies, and in those who caught respiratory infections, symptoms lasted less than half as long as in those taking a placebo (about 3.4 days, compared to 8.6 days).

Buy products that contain both *E. purpurea* and *E. angustifolia* species standardized to 4 percent echinacosides. Take echinacea at the first sign of a cold, but don't use it continuously for more than ten days. Take one dropperful of tincture in water four times a day, or two capsules of freeze-dried extract four times a day, or follow the package directions. Don't use echinacea if you have an autoimmune condition such as lupus or rheumatoid arthritis.

Use Elderberry for Colds to Feel Better, Faster

The antiviral and antibacterial herb elderberry (*Sambucus nigra*) is worth considering when it comes to revving up the immune system to reduce the symptoms and duration of colds and flu. Black elderberries are rich in anthocyanins, the active compounds in the fruit that provide the benefits. A study in *Nutrients* of 312 Australian passengers traveling overseas showed that taking Sambucol Elderberry Extract reduced the length and severity of cold symptoms. Researchers concluded that the extract activated immunity by boosting inflammatory cytokine production. Take elderberry in extracts, tinctures, teas, supplements, and lozenges. Follow package directions.

Powerful Habits to Turn Back the Clock on Your Sex Life

07

Just because you've taken a few more trips around the sun doesn't mean that your sex life needs to suffer. Being proactive and using tips, strategies, and new habits can help you move past obstacles and ensure many more years of satisfying sex.

Test your Sexual Health IQ here:

TRUE

FALSE

(T) (F) *The healthier you are as you get older, the more years of good sex you can have.*

(T) (F) *Positive self-esteem can boost your sex drive in later life.*

(T) (F) *Learning to be present in the moment isn't particularly important for intimacy as you get older.*

(T) (F) *It's worth it to make a commitment to exercising regularly because it improves your sex life in so many ways.*

(T) (F) *Stress doesn't significantly impact sexual problems such as erectile dysfunction (ED) and diminished desire.*

(T) (F) *After your twenties, your sex life will never be as good.*

(T) (F) *All supplements that claim to boost sex drive are largely unproven, usually ineffective, and sometimes even downright dangerous.*

HABIT #1
Address Underlying Health Issues for a Longer Love Life

The healthier you are as you get older, the more years of good sex you can have.
TRUE

Researchers looked at a group of 3,000 adults aged fifty-seven to eighty-five and, based on their survey responses, calculated that at age fifty-five, the sexually active life expectancy was 15 years for men and 10.6 years for women. They also found that men who were in very good or excellent health added on average five to seven years of active sexuality. For women in the study, being in very good shape added three to six more years of a superior sex life.

Health problems like arthritis or rheumatism, diabetes, high blood pressure, heart disease, and depression can all affect desire and sexual performance. While preventing these conditions in the first place is ideal, treating them or addressing the problematic symptoms can help you have satisfying sex for years to come.

Stiff, Sore Joints, or Chronic Pain

These conditions cause pain that can make sexual contact uncomfortable and interfere with intimacy. But there are solutions:

- *Try the tips in chapter 4 to keep your joints flexible and reduce pain, and experiment to see if sex is more comfortable for you at different times—in the morning or evening, after exercising, or after a warm bath, for example.*
- *Changing positions may also help. For example, try lying on your side, or having the partner with less pain on top.*
- *Some pain medications affect sexual function, so talk to your doctor if you think they're causing side effects.*

The Problem with Diabetes

Diabetes, and the obesity that usually accompanies it, can cause ED in some men. Researchers aren't as sure how diabetes affects women's sexuality, but a 2009 study in the *Journal of Sexual Medicine* found that diabetic women were more likely to have trouble reaching orgasm. Diabetes also increases the risk of vaginal yeast infections, which can make sex uncomfortable. Lifestyle changes, including eating a healthier diet, losing weight, and exercising, as well as drugs to control blood sugar can help restore sexual function in both men and women.

CHECK MEDICATION SIDE EFFECTS THAT AGE YOU SEXUALLY

A natural decline in hormone levels may make a difference in sexual response by midlife for both men and women. Complicating matters, health problems such as heart disease, atherosclerosis, high blood pressure, diabetes, and depression can also cause difficulties with arousal and orgasm, vaginal dryness, and ED. Many medications prescribed to treat the very conditions causing sexual complications can lower libido, weaken arousal, and make ED worse. Drugs for high blood pressure and depression are the worst culprits.

—

Blood pressure drugs. Diuretics dilate blood vessels and reduce fluid levels in the body, and beta-blockers act on your nervous system to counter stress-related spikes in blood pressure. Both have been shown to lower libido, contribute to ED in men, and delay orgasm in women.

Selective serotonin reuptake inhibitors (SSRIs). Untreated depression can cause sexual dysfunction. But research shows that SSRI antidepressants dampen desire, partly because of the way they affect neurotransmitters and other hormones and enzymes that impact your central nervous system. Instead, try mood boosters like exercise and social interaction to buoy your spirits, or even therapy, if you need it. You may be able to lower your dose of SSRIs or consider switching meds.

—

Statins have been linked to ED in men, and prescription or over-the-counter decongestants and antihistamines that dry up your runny nose can also increase vaginal dryness. If you're taking drugs for other conditions and experience sexual side effects, ask your doctor about other options.

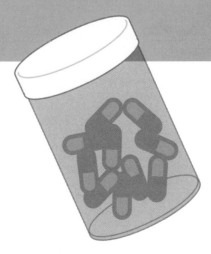

High Blood Pressure = Sexual Problems

About two-thirds of men with high blood pressure note problems with ED, and hypertension-related ED tends to be worse than in men with normal blood pressure. Women with hypertension are also more than twice as likely to report sexual dysfunction. Common hypertension drugs such as diuretics and beta-blockers can also have sexual side effects, such as lowered libido, ED, and delayed orgasm in women.

Switching drugs or lowering blood pressure through lifestyle changes can put the sizzle back into your sex life. Heart disease is linked to ED in men, and they share the same primary risk factors: high LDL ("bad") cholesterol, smoking, hypertension, and diabetes. Changes to blood vessels also reduce blood flow, which can cause both men and women to have trouble with orgasms. Most patients with stable heart conditions can safely be sexually active, and treatment for ED and to improve blood vessel health (such as controlling hypertension and cholesterol) can make sex more enjoyable.

> **MAKE IT A HABIT: IMPROVE HEALTH FOR BETTER SEX**
>
> Prevent or treat health problems such as arthritis, diabetes, high blood pressure, heart disease, and depression to add years to your sex life. Try natural treatments such as exercise and social interaction to control underlying conditions; medication side effects often include reduced desire or other sexual problems. If you're experiencing unwanted sexual side effects from medications, ask your doctor about other options.

HABIT #2
Maintain Sexual Confidence as You Age

Positive self-esteem can boost your sex drive in later life.
TRUE

Self-confidence is always sexy, no matter your age, and research shows that better body image can boost sex drive, even if you've noticed it dwindling over the years. For example, a 2009 study in the *Archives of Sexual Behavior* found that women who felt better about their bodies reported greater sexual desire. Feelings about sexual attractiveness and concern about weight—two factors the researchers used to measure body confidence—were most significantly related to desire, possibly because those aspects are most on display during sexual intimacy. So, cultivating a positive body image can pay off in the bedroom.

A 2024 study in *Psychology: Research and Review* showed a positive connection between women's self-esteem, sexual desire, and sexual assertiveness when it comes to sexual function. Other research shows that both sexes need positive sexual self-esteem to keep up their sexual desire in later life.

Self-confidence in general as you get older can ensure a more passionate love life for years to come. Women sixty-five and over who had high general self-esteem and stable partners had more sexual experiences than those who had neither. Some research shows that older adults have lower self-esteem, so it's worth working on for better sex and overall well-being. Try these tips to increase your own or your partner's self-confidence.

List Your Ageless, Lust-Worthy Qualities

Both bodies and life circumstances change over time, and what you used to take pride in (a flat stomach, work accomplishments) may no longer apply or have lost some luster. But rather than wishing you were twenty-five again, celebrate yourself as you are now to help restore your self-confidence and even refresh your romantic life. Here's how:

Make a list of ten things you like about yourself; compile it in your head or write it down to refer to when you need a lift. Include both physical attributes (strong shoulders, sparkling eyes) and character traits (generous, quick to laugh) that make you feel attractive.

You and your partner can create lists for each other as well— simply knowing that your partner finds you desirable can send your self-esteem soaring, and you might be surprised at what he or she finds alluring about you!

1 ....

2 ....

3 ....

4 ....

5 ....

6 ....

7 ....

8 ....

9 ....

10

Exercise Makes You Feel Sexy
No Matter Your Age

Of course, exercise can help you regain a youthful figure and increase sexy muscle definition, which may help you feel better about revealing your body in the bedroom. But exercise is also one of the best ways to increase your self-confidence regardless of your age or shape. A 2008 study in the *Journal of Physiology and Pharmacology* found that middle-aged, obese women who exercised at least twice a week for two months rated their appearance better than their non-exercising peers did, no matter their weight.

Exercise also increases blood flow to body parts involved in arousal and triggers the release of mood-boosting endorphins; both may spike your self-confidence and make you more willing to pursue a passionate encounter with your partner.

Do Something You're Good at
to Feel Sexually Attractive

Because it tends to strongly influence your sense of identity, self-esteem, and self-worth in all areas of life—including your sexuality—it's worth making sure you enjoy your occupation or avocation, note researchers in a 2009 study in the *Journal of Women's Health and Gender-Based Medicine*.

That may mean seeking extra responsibility at work, starting a new business, volunteering, renewing friendships, or making more time for a hobby. Any activity that allows you to excel will reward you with greater self-confidence, whether or not you receive recognition for your efforts. That renewed sense of self-worth can spill over into the bedroom. Likewise, seeing your partner shine can be a turn-on.

MAKE IT A HABIT:
SEXY SELF-CONFIDENCE

Make a list of ten things you like about yourself, including physical attributes and character traits.

Exercise to release endorphins, feel better about yourself, and boost blood flow to sexual body parts.

Do work you enjoy and pursue your hobbies; your success in these endeavors will lead to greater self-esteem.

HABIT# 3
Practice Mindfulness to Renew Romance

Learning to be present in the moment isn't particularly important for intimacy as you get older.
FALSE

Although it can enhance your love life at any age, learning to be present in the moment is particularly important for intimacy as you get older. For one thing, it can help short-circuit bedroom boredom, especially if you've been with your partner for a long time. Tuning in to the physical sensations and emotional aspects of sex can renew your feelings of closeness and make it more enjoyable. Research shows that women with mindfulness training reported that it significantly increased their desire and reduced their sexual distress, while helping them get aroused more easily.

> **WHAT IS MINDFULNESS?**
>
> Human minds tend to run all day long. The mind is always telling stories, good and bad, judging and ruminating, regretting and futurizing. Mindfulness is the conscious choice to slow down and focus on the now. When we do, there is an expansiveness to life that doesn't exist when we are running from task to task or moment to moment without paying real attention to what is going on. Choosing to cultivate the habit of mindfulness and becoming more aware changes all that and enables you to be in the present moment, which can make life more manageable (less reacting and overwhelm, more being), and pleasurable experiences, including sex, more enjoyable.

Master Your Mind for Better Sex

Mindfulness practices and a non-goal-oriented approach to sex can take pressure off and even help you redefine what makes a satisfying sexual experience. Evidence indicates that as people get older, they're not able to climax as easily as they used to. But you can still enjoy the ride, so to speak.

A review of studies suggests relieving the pressure of performance may be one reason why yoga, which means centering yourself in the now, can help treat premature ejaculation in men. Likewise, it may be why mindfulness practices improve several aspects of sexual response and reduce sexual distress in women with desire and arousal disorders, which are more common the older you get.

When you're distracted, it's harder to be in the moment and respond sexually. Meditation and other mindfulness practices help you change this and enjoy the present. A 2014 study in *Behaviour Research and Therapy* that focused on group mindfulness training with women over a four-week period showed improvement in sexual desire, arousal, and satisfaction. Six months later, participants reported continued positive effects from the training.

Learning to be more mindful doesn't take a lot of effort—it simply involves slowing down and paying closer attention to your surroundings. If setting aside fifteen minutes to practice mindfulness as part of meditation appeals to you, go for it. But you can also reap the benefits by sneaking in a few mindful moments here and there.

Start Outside the Bedroom

You may find it easier to begin in a nonsexual setting. Use all your senses to observe the world around you, such as the smell of a candle or the sound of a clock ticking. When it's comfortable, try applying that to sex—think about what kissing tastes like, the feel of your skin on the sheets, the smell of your partner's hair. Noticing these details can help you reclaim your desire for and enjoyment of sex. By helping you appreciate little things about your partner, it may even restore a spark if your love life has settled into routine.

Yoga for Mindfulness

Yoga provides the dual benefits of exercise and mindfulness because many of the poses involve balance and focusing on your breath. Maintaining your balance demands concentration—just try standing on one leg while you're mentally rehashing your to-do list—and taking deep breaths or breathing in a pattern requires some thought. A 2009 study in the *Journal of Sexual Medicine* found that after practicing yoga for twelve weeks, women rated several aspects of sexual function (desire, arousal, lubrication, orgasm, satisfaction, and pain) better than at the start of the study.

> **MAKE IT A HABIT: MINDFUL SEXUALITY**
>
> Practice mindfulness daily by staying present in the moment, rather than allowing your mind to race or wander. Be aware of the sensations of physical intimacy: the sight of your partner's body, the smell of his hair, the touch of skin upon skin. Stretch or practice yoga to loosen your body while focusing your mind. Use sight, scent, and touch to improve foreplay and sex.

ENLIST ALL YOUR SENSES TO RESTORE YOUTHFUL DESIRE

Mindfulness also helps you pay attention to all of your senses. Appealing to all of them pays off in increased interest in sexual activity, easier arousal, better performance, and overall greater enjoyment in lovemaking—all things that often decline as you get older. So, it's definitely worth the effort.

—

Sight. Good grooming is a must and lingerie helps, but you should also clear visual clutter from your bedroom to reduce distraction and make your bed with your nicest linens. Brush your teeth or pop a mint to make kissing more fun. Put on some mood music, whether you prefer Frank Sinatra, Barry White, or classic rock. All of this sends romantic cues to your brain that help set the stage for intimacy.

—

Smell. Scent can be a powerful aphrodisiac. Aromatherapy using lavender essential oil (four drops of essential oil diluted with 20 ml of hot water and inhaled for thirty minutes) noticeably reduced cortisol levels and improved blood flow in male volunteers in a 2008 study in the *International Journal of Cardiology*. Better blood flow is linked to superior sexual performance for both men and women. Lavender also acts on the autonomic nervous system, which includes the parasympathetic nerves, to simultaneously induce relaxation and increase arousal.

—

Touch. A hug, holding hands, and a caress on the cheek are all simple ways to show your affection for your partner, and touching, even in ways that aren't explicitly sexual, can increase arousal. Skin-to-skin contact triggers the release of oxytocin, a powerful hormone that enhances feelings of love and desire. Extended foreplay can liven up your lovemaking and increases lubrication for older women with vaginal dryness, making for a more passionate encounter for both partners. You can also experiment with water-based lubricants to make sexual touch more pleasurable.

Notably, women over age forty-five reported more improvement than the younger volunteers did. A 2010 study in the same journal showed that yoga improved many aspects of sexual function, including satisfaction, performance, and confidence.

While yoga has a long tradition of benefiting sexuality, regularly performing any kind of stretching and balance exercises will offer similar effects as long as you treat them as an opportunity to focus your attention. You can also stretch with your partner, allowing you to connect with each other in a different, but still physical, way.

HABIT #4
Exercise to Reverse Age-Related Sexual Problems

It's worth it to make a commitment to exercising regularly because it improves your sex life in so many ways.
TRUE

Exercise gives you energy, relieves stress, triggers the release of mood-boosting endorphins, helps you reconnect with your body, improves health conditions that can interfere with sex, and can help you lose weight and feel more confident. It also increases blood flow, muscle tone, and agility, all of which decline with age but are critical for arousal and performance, balance, and being able to hold sexual positions comfortably.

A study in *Sexual Medicine Reviews* in 2018 noted that, for women, exercise contributes to a positive body image, which can mean better sex. They also found that exercise improves sexual arousal due to a boost in sympathetic nervous system and endocrine activity. Exercise can also help with lower libido and ED, common problems for men that come with aging.

Start with Aerobic Exercise for Better Sex as You Age

Any kind of activity that gets your heart pumping will boost blood flow to all parts of your body, including your genitals, which can increase arousal and lead to better sexual performance. In fact, improvement in blood vessel health is one reason why exercise is so effective in treating ED.

Try to do at least thirty minutes of exercise a day on most days of the week. Breaking it up into ten-minute chunks will still benefit your body if that's the only way you can squeeze it in, but try to make a few of your sessions longer to increase your endurance and keep your blood vessels young and healthy.

> **MAKE IT A HABIT: EXERCISE FOR SEX**
>
> Exercise increases blood flow, muscle tone, and sexual agility, while releasing feel-good hormones and helping you lose weight. Get your heart pumping with aerobic exercise to counteract low libido and ED. Do Kegels and consistent strength training to restore desire and improve sexual function. Lift weights to boost testosterone production.

LIFT WEIGHTS TO BOOST LOW TESTOSTERONE

With age, levels of the sex hormone testosterone decrease in both men and women, which may be why older adults tend to have a lower sex drive and report more sexual problems. Low testosterone levels are likely responsible for lowered libido and ED in some men. Women produce testosterone in their ovaries, and levels decline—along with estrogen—during menopause. Strength training in particular can build muscle strength and stimulate the release of testosterone. Aim for twenty to thirty minutes of strength training two or three times a week, working all of your major muscle groups, and giving your muscles a day to rest in between sessions. To continue increasing your testosterone levels, you need to switch up your moves, the intensity, and reps you do—keep pushing yourself.

Step Up Your Strength Training for More Confident Lovemaking

Resistance exercise, whether you use weights, elastic bands, or your own body weight, increases muscle tone and strength—and that can enhance your sexual response and ability. It can also help you feel more confident with your clothes off: University of Houston researchers found that as little as six weeks of strength training significantly improved how men and women rated their appearance and body satisfaction. To build muscle, do strength exercises twice a week on nonconsecutive days for thirty minutes or more. Be sure to work all your major muscle groups: chest, upper and lower back, shoulders and arms, quadriceps (quads) and hips, hamstrings and glutes, calves, and abdominal muscles.

Kegels: Good for Women and Men

In addition to traditional strength moves, Kegels, exercises that target your pelvic floor muscles, can increase pleasure and sexual satisfaction in women, since pregnancy and childbirth can weaken those muscles. But aging also affects pelvic floor muscles—in both men and women. That means Kegels can actually benefit men as well. Kegels increase blood flow and muscle tone to pelvic floor muscles, which improve vaginal intercourse. For both men and women, they can help prevent urinary incontinence down the road.

To do a Kegel, tighten your pelvic muscles as if you were stopping the flow of urine. For sexual benefits, do ten Kegels several times a day for eight to twelve weeks. Remember, just like any other strength exercise, you have to keep it up to maintain the benefits!

HABIT #5
Dial Back Stress to Rev Up Your Love Life

Stress doesn't significantly impact sexual problems such as ED and diminished desire.

FALSE

Too much stress and tension can exacerbate the sexual problems that older adults commonly face, such as ED and diminished desire. Stress can also make you tired because it activates the fight-or-flight response, which triggers a cortisol release. Cortisol makes you ready for action or to flee, but when it wears off fatigue can result. Learning how to manage and lower stress levels and getting enough rest can make a significant difference in sexual problems, putting the spark back into your sex life today and helping you stay sexually satisfied well into later life.

Stop Mid- and Late-Life Stress from Sapping Your Desire

In addition to everyday stresses, older adults face some uniquely challenging situations, such as retirement, illness, caring for aging parents, and other lifestyle adjustments. Piling stress upon stress may lead to sexual difficulties and strain your relationship. A 2008 population study found that for men and women aged fifty-seven to eighty-five, stress and anxiety were linked to several sexual problems, including lack of interest, inability to orgasm, pain during sex, lack of pleasure in sex, and worries about performance. Women noted that tension worsened vaginal dryness as well, while men additionally reported trouble achieving and maintaining an erection and climaxing too early.

Stress can also be caused relationship dissatisfaction, while being happy with your relationship is associated with higher sexual pleasure, increased ability to orgasm for women, and greater sexual interest for men. If you have unresolved relationship problems, consider seeing a therapist to help you work through your issues and restore emotional intimacy.

The pressure to perform sexually can reduce sex drive and trigger ED in men too. By age sixty-five, between 15 and 25 percent of men experience impotence, or ED, at least one out of every four times they have sex. Talk to your doctor about treating health conditions, lifestyle changes, medications, and other strategies that can improve ED.

Fight Fatigue for Better Sex Year after Year

Fatigue depletes your sex drive, and the older you get, the more likely you are to have trouble sleeping thanks to medications, shifting hormones, changing responsibilities, and chronic conditions. But being well rested can restore your libido. To get your forty winks:

- *Dedicate enough time for sleep.*

- *Avoid eating, drinking caffeine, or doing anything stimulating (other than sex) right before bed.*

- *Reduce or eliminate alcohol. Alcohol interferes with sleep. It can also numb your sex drive, cause erection problems in men, and delay orgasm in women.*

- *Keep your bedroom dark and quiet, and set a regular sleep schedule.*

- *Ask your doctor if medications or health problems might be interfering with your sleep, and whether switching drugs or reducing the dose, lifestyle changes, or alternative therapies could help treat the underlying condition without the sleep-stealing side effects.*

Change Up Your Routine

If you're exhausted, it can be hard to pursue a passionate moment. But, once you get started, you'll enjoy it and end up with more energy afterward. Try having sex at the times of day when you have the most get-up-and-go, whether that's first thing in the morning or after a workout. See the tips in chapter 8 for more ideas on how to raise your energy levels enough to fuel an active sex life.

**MAKE IT A HABIT:
REDUCE STRESS FOR BETTER SEX**

Dedicate enough time for sleep and avoid eating, drinking caffeine, or doing anything stimulating (other than sex) right before bed.

Don't drink to sleep or relieve stress; alcohol can numb your sex drive.

See a therapist if you are overwhelmed by stressors common to older people: retirement, caring for aged parents, illness, and so on, or if you have unresolved relationship tension.

HABIT #6
Be Honest about Shifting Needs and Desires

After your twenties, your sex life will never be as good.
FALSE

Just because things don't work like they did when you were in your twenties doesn't mean you can't have passionate, fulfilling sex. For example, in a group of women between the ages of forty-five and eighty, an average of 43 percent reported having at least moderate sexual desire, and half of the sexually active participants described their overall sexual satisfaction as moderate to high, according to a 2009 study in the *Journal of the American Geriatrics Society*. Around 60 to 70 percent of men in that age range also reported moderate to high sexual desire in a 2005 study in the *Journal of Sex Research*.

Staying in good overall health can help you maintain an active, healthy sex life for longer. Understanding natural changes in desire, arousal, and satisfaction can help you accept them and adapt your lovemaking to ease sexual difficulties and explore new aspects of your sexuality. Talking openly with your partner is also critical, especially so he or she doesn't misinterpret physical changes as a lack of interest.

Learn about Physical Changes as You Age

Talk to your doctor about how aging, illnesses, menopause, and medications might affect your sex life. Knowing how your body (and your partner's) works and what is a healthy sexual response can ease anxiety. For example, men's testosterone levels decline with age, which can lead to lower libido, needing more time and stimulation for erection and orgasm, shorter orgasms, and taking longer to achieve another erection after ejaculation.

Women might notice more vaginal dryness, lower desire, or that hot flashes are keeping them up at night and leaving them exhausted (and not exactly in the mood) during the day. Confide in your partner about whatever changes you're experiencing and find ways of being intimate that both of you can enjoy.

PRACTICE NONSEXUAL INTIMACY TO EXTEND YOUR SEX LIFE

"Age does not protect you from love. But love, to some extent, protects you from age," said actress Jeanne Moreau. Put another way, if you want to stay young, you need to nurture the love in your life. These habits can help:

Restore emotional closeness. Return to the early days of your relationship—learning about your partner's likes and dislikes, hopes, and dreams for the future. Those kinds of conversations, rather than the logistics of daily life, build intimacy and can restore that sexual spark. You may be surprised at how each of you has changed. Ask, and really listen to the answers. Open communication builds trust.

Make dates. Setting aside time for just the two of you cultivates closeness, but it also communicates that your partner is a priority, that you don't take him or her for granted even if you've been together forever, and that your relationship is important enough to nurture.

Express your love and appreciation. Pay attention, compliment, and express appreciation for things your partner does.

Resolve conflicts that make you feel distant; consider couples therapy. A skilled counselor can help you navigate sources of tension and learn how to fight fair. Your therapist may also have suggestions for how to meet each other's emotional needs.

Enjoy nonsexual touch. With skin-on-skin contact, you experience a rush of the "love hormone" oxytocin. A 2008 study in the journal *Psychosomatic Medicine* found that couples assigned to a "warm touch" intervention (including hugging, massage, and other physical displays of affection) for four weeks had higher levels of oxytocin. Snuggle, offer a goodbye kiss, and welcome your partner home with a hug.

Use It or Lose It

Having sex regularly makes it easier and more enjoyable to continue having sex as you get older. As women go through menopause and their estrogen levels drop, the vaginal walls become thinner and less elastic. However, sexual activity that involves penetration can slow or even reverse this process. For men, going for a long time without an erection can lower blood flow to the penis and reduce the muscle cells' ability to expand when blood flow does increase, making it harder to achieve and maintain an erection. But having sex regularly boosts circulation to the genitals, increasing both pleasure and sexual function.

Discuss Concerns and Wants for Lifelong Satisfaction

Good communication is essential for all aspects of a healthy relationship, including sex. Discuss your concerns, write down your thoughts and share them, or read a book about sexuality together and underline passages that appeal to you. Seek out a professional counselor who can help you understand what's normal and suggest ways to share your feelings about sex with your partner. Ultimately, being honest can bring you closer to your partner and help you both enjoy sex and intimacy more.

Try Something New to Refresh a Stale Sex Life

Keeping your romantic life fresh and fun is one way to maintain sexual desire and increase satisfaction as you get older, especially if you've been with your partner for years. Monotony in sexual relationships, such as predictability of sexual activities and over-familiarity with the partner, may contribute to a loss in sexual desire.

Boredom undermines closeness but novelty boosts the brain chemical dopamine, according to University College London researchers. Dopamine is linked to the brain's reward center and helps fuel sex drive, and studies show that all kinds of new experiences, images, people, and thoughts can trigger its release.

Try a new activity—and it doesn't have to be sexual. This can be anything from visiting a museum to exploring an unfamiliar walking path together or playing pickleball. Celebrating milestones and achievements also cultivates closeness and can rekindle a spark. Wearing sexy lingerie, sharing fantasies, role-playing, using sex toys or lubricants, and attempting new positions can all help you break out of a sexual rut. Be adventurous and use your imagination and you may just find an incredibly pleasurable new favorite!

MAKE IT A HABIT: TALK OPENLY FOR BETTER SEX AND BE OPEN TO NEW EXPERIENCES

Honesty sparks intimacy: Discuss your physical and emotional changes with your partner. Older men might need more time and stimulation for erection and orgasm; older women might experience vaginal dryness, lower desire, and hot flashes at night that disrupt sleep and leave them wiped out.

Use it or lose it! Intercourse can slow the thinning of the vaginal walls, and men who go without an erection for an extended period of time may find it harder to achieve one. Be willing to try new things with your partner in and out of the bedroom to reinvigorate your sex life.

NEEDS AND WANTS

HABIT #7
Take Herbs and Supplements to Reignite a Sexual Spark

All supplements that claim to boost sex drive are largely unproven, usually ineffective, and sometimes even downright dangerous.
FALSE

Research-backed supplements can help revive a waning libido, improve ED, and relieve other age-related sexual problems. Always talk to your doctor before taking supplements, natural or not, since many interact with medications or other herbs, or may not be safe to take if you have certain health conditions.

ArginMax Increases Sexual Satisfaction

This proprietary supplement combines the amino acid L-arginine and the herbs ginkgo, ginseng, and damiana, plus vitamins and minerals, to increase desire and improve sexual function. Your body uses L-arginine to make nitric oxide, which relaxes blood vessels and boosts blood flow. Ginkgo has a similar effect. Besides increasing nitric oxide levels, ginseng acts as a mild stimulant and sexual "energizer." Damiana (*Turnera diffusa*) may calm anxiety and is a reputed aphrodisiac, but it hasn't been well studied.

Women going through menopause who took the supplement reported having more sex, having higher sexual desire and being more satisfied with their sexual relationship, as well as having better vaginal lubrication, compared to women taking a placebo, noted a 2006 study in the *Journal of Sex and Marital Therapy*. In a small study investigating ArginMax in men, almost all the volunteers said they were better able to maintain an erection during intercourse, and 75 percent were more satisfied with their sex life. Men's and women's formulations are available; follow package directions for dosing. Allow four weeks to notice a difference. The supplement seems to be safe—no studies have reported significant side effects.

Give Ginkgo and Ginseng a Try to Improve Arousal

Ginkgo biloba facilitates blood flow and relaxes smooth muscle tissue while enhancing the effects of nitric oxide, helping men achieve and maintain an erection. In a 2008 *Archives of Sexual Behavior* study, women taking ginkgo for eight weeks along with sex therapy noted greater sexual desire and contentment compared to placebo. Some evidence suggests it may benefit people experiencing sexual side effects from antidepressants. The usual amount is 120 milligrams daily, in divided doses with food. It's relatively safe, although you shouldn't use it while taking blood thinners. The active compounds in Asian ginseng (*Panax ginseng*), called *ginsenosides,* increase nitric oxide and relax blood vessels and expandable tissues in the penis that fill with blood during an erection. Men taking ginseng reported better erectile function and overall satisfaction after eight weeks, researchers noted in the *Asian Journal of Andrology*. Search for standardized extracts and follow package dosing directions; allow six to eight weeks to see an effect. Ginseng is generally considered safe, but it can raise blood pressure and cause irritability and insomnia in some people.

Beneficial Vitamins for Men's Sexual Health

A review of studies in the *International Journal for Vitamin and Nutrition Research* in 2023 showed that supplementing with *niacin (B3)* 1500 milligrams daily for 12 weeks improved ED due to a boost in blood flow. Food sources of B3 include meat, fish, and poultry along with whole and fortified grains. A 1996 study in *Nutrition* showed that serum testosterone levels were affected by *zinc* levels. Find zinc in beef, oysters, and fish. A 2018 study in the *International Journal of Impotence Research* showed that low levels of *vitamin D* can negatively impact sexual function. You'll find vitamin D in fatty fish and fortified dairy products like milk. If you want to supplement with these vitamins, check with your health care practitioner, especially if you have a medical condition.

Revive a Waning Libido with Maca

Maca (*Lepidium meyenii*), a Peruvian root traditionally used as an aphrodisiac, may improve desire and sexual function, and in turn, your general sense of well-being. Men with mild ED who took maca for twelve weeks reported better erections and feeling happier with their sex lives than men taking a placebo, according to a 2009 study in *Andrologia*. Postmenopausal women taking maca for six weeks reported less anxiety and depression and a nearly 35 percent improvement in sexual problems compared to placebo, noted a 2008 study in *Menopause*. Maca seems to be well tolerated and has few side effects. Studies used between 1.5 and 3.5 grams, with 3 grams daily considered a high, but safe and effective, dose.

Powerful Habits to Turn Back the Clock for More Energy

08

Boosting energy levels is one of the most important things you can do to feel younger and be able to do more. But many things can sap energy and make you feel fatigued. How much do you know about how to boost and sustain energy so you can do all the things you really want to do?

Check your Energy IQ here >

TRUE

FALSE

T   F   *Chronic stress can make you feel tired.*

T   F   *Being inactive stores up energy so that you have it when you need it.*

T   F   *Eating simple sugars is fine because it gives you short bursts of energy when you need it.*

T   F   *Caffeine gives you energy, but eating a healthy diet and, if needed, supplementing with important vitamins and minerals, gives you more long-lasting results.*

T   F   *Once you reach mid or late life, it's best to conserve energy rather than trying to find purpose.*

HABIT #1
Don't Let Stress Slow You Down

Chronic stress can make you feel tired.
TRUE

Stress can send already-flagging energy levels into a downward spiral. Chronic tension can wear you out—exposure to continuously high levels of stress hormones such as cortisol keep your body in a fight-or-flight response that it just can't maintain long term, and your energy levels pay the price. Here's how to dial down and put the pep back in your step.

Do One Thing at a Time

The first order of business is to take care of your health: Eat well, exercise regularly, and get enough sleep. These basics are increasingly important as your natural energy production slows over time. Next, center yourself in the moment and stop trying to do too many things at once. You may think that multitasking helps you be more efficient with your time, and to some extent—like washing the dishes while talking on the phone or listening to a book on tape during your commute—that can be true.

But trying to do more than one task that requires similar levels of attention, like paying bills while talking on the phone, means that neither gets your full concentration. A 2014 study in *Stress and Health: Journal of the International Society for the Investigation of Stress* showed that multitasking actually increased heart rate and blood pressure. So, it may also not be good for your health.

Ultimately, multitasking takes longer to do both because you're constantly breaking focus to switch between them, which can skew your perception of how much you actually have to do, unnecessarily increasing stress and making you feel frazzled. You'll be more productive and focused if you organize tasks into time chunks of an hour or two and switch to a new task after that.

Identify the time-stealers that you frequently try to tack on to other tasks. If that's email or Facebook, for example, set aside specific times to check your inbox and respond (twice a day, once an hour, and so on). That frees you to devote complete attention to a job and do it well so you can cross it off your to-do list and move on.

Get Organized

Organizing your time can help calm the anxiety of feeling overwhelmed and lift the sense of overarching dread that so often accompanies it. Instead of letting monster projects—from your company's annual report to your parents' golden wedding anniversary party—hang over your head and drain you, control the chaos by breaking them down into manageable chunks and tackling them one by one.

Try using apps for daily planning or go analog and try a bullet journal to create monthly and daily logs to help you prioritize and complete tasks.

Have Fun Every Day to Live a More Fulfilling Life

Another key to relieving energy-sapping stress as you get older is to make time for things you enjoy. Even if you only have a few minutes, taking a walk outside, reading a chapter in a good book, or calling a friend can refresh your spirits and your energy levels. Inject fun into your life whenever you can for a natural lift: Tell jokes to your coworkers, juggle your groceries as you put them away, listen to music while you do chores. Learn relaxation skills such as deep breathing techniques, guided imagery, and meditation that you can use to unwind whenever you need a moment of peace.

Humor may provide extra stress-squashing benefits, whether you watch a classic comedy or listen to a friend regale you with a sidesplitting anecdote. "Laughter releases excessive physical and psychological energy, and it reduces stress, anxiety, worry, and frustration," note the authors of a study in the *Journal of Gerontological Nursing*. If you find yourself fretting over factors out of your control, seek out witty friends who can divert your attention and help you regain perspective. Besides making difficult situations seem more manageable, the social support busts stress by giving you a safe outlet to share concerns and get feedback—and you'll likely return to the problem with a fresh approach and renewed energy.

> **MAKE IT A HABIT: STRESS RELIEVERS**
>
> Stop trying to do so much at once. Multitasking actually makes you less effective, not more. Take the time to do the things you enjoy. Spend time outdoors or with a friend, or pair not-so-fun activities (such as chores) with more enjoyable pursuits such as listening to your favorite music. Laugh more. Watch comedies, go to comedy clubs, and call a witty friend to help you see things in a new light and lighten your stress load.

HABIT #2
Use Newton's Law: Keep Moving to Counteract Fatigue

Being inactive stores up energy so that you have it when you need it.

FALSE

Newton's first law of motion states, in part, that an object at rest tends to stay at rest. That applies to your body too—the longer you're inactive, the more sluggish you'll feel, and the harder it can be to motivate yourself to move. But the opposite also applies: Increasing your daily activity can send your energy levels skyrocketing.

> **INSTANT ENERGY!**
>
> For instant invigoration, drink a glass of cold water, or if you're brave, give yourself a quick blast of cold water in the shower. Splash cold water on your face, or gargle with it—the sudden temperature change shakes off morning fogginess. You can also give yourself an invigorating rubdown with a washcloth or loofah to get your blood flowing (use a body wash or soap with an energizing scent for extra help waking up). Mint-flavored toothpaste can also give you a subtle boost by acting on a nerve in your brain that helps you feel more energized.

Don't Mix Up Mental and Physical Fatigue

You may feel wiped out after sitting at a desk all day, but it's easy to confuse being mentally tired with being physically tired. After about forty-five minutes of inactivity, you'll start to feel fatigued. But you can break out of that sedentary stupor just by getting up from your chair. Physical movement is invigorating because it boosts circulation and loosens tight muscles and joints (both of which get worse with age), and it gives your cells a burst of energizing oxygen. Take advantage of those benefits by adding movement throughout your day, especially to break up monotonous tasks or long periods of sitting, or at times when you normally feel like a zombie.

ADD EXTRA ACTIVITY TO YOUR ROUTINE

Older adults stand and walk less per day than younger people do, according to a 2007 study in the *American Journal of Physiology: Endocrinology and Metabolism*. The researchers suggested that lean, healthy older adults may actually "have a biological drive to be less active than the young." So, in addition to your daily workout, it's important to find ways to add extra activity to your normal routine:

- *Pace while you're on the phone.*
- *Conduct walking meetings at work.*
- *Eat at your desk and take a quick walk around the block during your lunch break.*
- *Swap your chair for a stability ball (you have to use your leg and core muscles to keep yourself balanced, and you can also bounce on it from time to time).*

The more you move, the more energetic you'll feel. As a bonus, moving more throughout your day can rev up a sluggish midlife metabolism, helping you lose weight and making it even easier to be active. It also ensures you'll be able to stay active well into late life.

Fight Fatigue with Exercise

Regular low and moderate-intensity exercise can combat fatigue, according to a 2008 study in the journal *Psychotherapy and Psychosomatics*. Sedentary but otherwise healthy volunteers who complained of constant tiredness reported significantly more energy after exercising for just twenty minutes three times a week for six weeks. What's more, each exerciser reported at least a 49 percent drop in feelings of fatigue. Strength training provides similar benefits.

And while you should aim for at least thirty minutes of exercise on most days of the week for good overall health, research shows that even a few minutes of low-intensity movement here and there can stimulate your central nervous system, clearing out mental cobwebs and helping you feel more alert.

HABIT #3
Eat to Sustain All-Day Energy

Eating simple sugars is fine because it gives you short bursts of energy when you need it.
FALSE

Eating energy-stabilizing foods can help revive flagging energy levels. Your body—especially your brain, which has few energy reserves of its own—needs a steady supply of blood sugar to function at its best, but too much or too little can leave you drained. Filling up on simple carbs or going too long without eating can weaken your body's response to insulin, the hormone that helps you use glucose (sugar) for energy. Besides sapping your strength, over time insulin resistance can cause high levels of glucose to build up in your blood and set the stage for diabetes, which speeds up aging throughout your body.

Fortunately, the foods that keep your blood sugar steady also provide nutrients necessary for energy-producing reactions in the body. Rich in vitamins, minerals, and antiaging antioxidants, this fountain-of-youth fare can restore energy, reduce your risk of age-accelerating diabetes, keep your waistline in check as you get older (see chapter 2), and ensure your body can operate at peak form for years to come.

Eat Right to Fuel Your Body Throughout the Day

Most people need to eat every three to four hours to avoid running on empty. Here's what to keep in mind:

Start the day the right way. Ditch the frosted cornflakes and lift your a.m. fog with a power breakfast of old-fashioned or steel-cut oats, milk, blueberries, pecans, and a sprinkle of blood sugar–lowering cinnamon.

Trim down your lunch. Having a large or high-carb lunch can exacerbate the afternoon slump triggered by your circadian rhythms, so downsize your portions and be sure to include protein, fat, and fiber to keep you going strong all afternoon. Make your lunch sandwich on 100 percent whole-wheat bread, add cucumbers and roasted red peppers to your lettuce and tomato, and trade your mayo for fiber- and protein-rich hummus.

Eat a Mediterranean diet dinner. For example, choose brown rice for your stir-fry, use a small amount of slow-burning lean protein, double the vegetables, and hold the sugary sauce.

Snack the right way. It's tempting to reach for a soda or cookies for a quick energy boost, but you'll crash just as swiftly. Instead, select snacks that combine protein, complex carbohydrates, and healthy fats for long-lasting energy—your body digests them steadily. Fiber-rich foods help lower insulin levels and slow the release of sugars into your blood. Recharge with snacks such as whole-grain crackers and cheese, fruit and nuts, plain yogurt with berries and granola, baby carrots and white bean dip, and celery and peanut butter.

Reach for Water to Boost Energy

Even mild dehydration can make you feel tired as you get older, so water should be the first beverage you reach for if you want to perk up. If you aren't hydrated enough, your body fluids can actually thicken slightly, which slows circulation and chemical reactions that produce energy throughout your body, according to a 2007 study in the *Journal of the American College of Nutrition*.

How much water you need depends on several factors, including your activity level and climate. Food (especially water-rich fruits and vegetables) can account for about 20 percent of your total fluid intake, according to the Mayo Clinic. In addition to diet, the Institute of Medicine suggests that men consume about thirteen cups (3 L) and women consume about nine cups (2.2 L) of total beverages a day. A good general guideline is that if you feel thirsty or notice your mouth is dry, start sipping.

Drink Green or Black Tea

If you need a caffeine boost, opt for green or black tea instead of coffee. Although tea doesn't contain as much caffeine per cup (only 20 to 30 milligrams in 8 ounces [240 ml], compared to 100 milligrams in coffee), it has the added benefits of powerful age-fighting antioxidants and stimulants like theophylline and the amino acid L-theanine, which can increase blood circulation, improve oxygen flow, and help you stay alert without feeling jittery. Green and black tea also help insulin regulate your blood sugar more effectively, preventing energy spikes and crashes and reducing your risk of developing type 2 diabetes.

MAKE IT A HABIT: EAT AND DRINK FOR ENERGY

Eat small snacks every three to four hours or so to keep your blood sugar steady. Combine protein with complex carbohydrates, such as peanut butter and apples or yogurt and granola.

Drink plenty of water to improve your circulation. For an energy boost, choose green or black tea over coffee for their antiaging antioxidants.

HABIT #4
Perk Up with Safe Supplements and Practices to Feel Younger

Caffeine gives you energy, but eating a healthy diet and, if needed, supplementing with important vitamins and minerals, gives you more long-lasting results.
TRUE

Yes, caffeine and related stimulants will give you a lift. However, another class of energy-enhancing supplements may revive waning energy levels as you get older without the jittery side effects. Derived from substances already in our bodies or that we get from food, these compounds affect how the body metabolizes the nutrients we eat and translates them into energy, studies show. If you get enough from a healthy, well-balanced diet, popping a pill probably won't help.

But if you're deficient because of poor eating habits, strenuous exercise, chronic stress, or regularly taking certain medications (such as acid blockers, anti-inflammatory painkillers, or antibiotics), supplementing might provide some benefit. Keep in mind, however, that lifestyle changes are likely to be far more effective than a supplement. Before taking these or any supplements, talk to your doctor about how they might affect any medical conditions you have and possible drug interactions.

Boost Flagging Energy with B Vitamins

B vitamins play an important role in energy production, helping you think clearly and improving sleep quality—and a deficiency makes you feel sluggish. For example, thiamin, or B1, helps nervous system tissue use blood tissue use blood sugar (glucose) to produce energy, and it plays a role in cognitive performance, especially in older adults. And vitamins B6 and B12, among others, are required to synthesize certain energizing neurotransmitters.

> **MAKE IT A HABIT: ENERGY-BOOSTING SUPPLEMENTS**
>
> Adults over fifty should take a B-50 complex supplement or a multivitamin with 100 percent of the RDA for B vitamins daily. Try ashwagandha root extract for stress and fatigue. Short-term use is safe; check first with your doctor if you have a medical condition. Try CoQ10 to relieve physical fatigue and make workouts seem easier. Tyrosine increases mental energy and alertness, but people with melanoma or phenylketonuria shouldn't take it.

FEEL YOUNGER WITH AROMATHERAPY

Along with supplements, natural practices like aromatherapy can relieve depression, anxiety, and stress, all of which sap energy and leave you lethargic. Certain scents are invigorating and immediately help you feel more alert. Try a few and find out which you like best.

—

Soothe energy-sapping stress with essential oils. Research indicates the most popular scents to ease anxiety include lavender (*Lavandula angustifolia*), rose (*Rosa damascena*), orange (*Citrus sinensis*), bergamot (*Citrus aurantium*), lemon (*Citrus limon*), sandalwood (*Santalum album*), clary sage (*Salvia sclarea*), Roman chamomile (*Anthemis nobilis*), and rose-scented geranium (*Pelargonium* spp.). Which scent, or combination, you choose to help you destress and energize is largely a matter of personal preference.

__ Smelling lavender essential oil lowers cortisol levels and boosts your body's free radical–scavenging activity, protecting you from aging, according to a 2007 study in *Psychiatry Research*.

__ Bergamot essential oil may also help minimize symptoms of stress-induced anxiety and mild mood disorders. Although researchers aren't sure exactly how it works, evidence suggests it acts on nerve tissue and protects the brain, notes a 2010 study in the journal *Fitoterapia*.

—

Perk up with stimulating scents. Research shows that peppermint (*Mentha piperita*), rosemary (*Rosmarinus officinalis*), jasmine (*Jasminum* spp.), and eucalyptus (*Eucalyptus globulus*) essential oils can erase fatigue. Peppermint essential oil increases alertness and memory. Rosemary essential oil lowers anxiety and, like jasmine, boosts alertness. Choose your favorite to offset flagging energy levels. Dilute and sprinkle drops on your pillow, burn candles, or keep a bottle handy and take a sniff as needed.

While most people get enough from food, it's common to fall below the RDAs for vitamin B6 and folate. As you get older, your body is also less able to absorb vitamin B12. Stress depletes the B vitamins as well, and many medications (such as acid blockers, antibiotics, or the antidiabetes drug Metformin) can interfere with absorption. Experts recommend that all adults over fifty take a B-50 complex supplement daily (which provides 50 milligrams of most of the B vitamins, plus 400 micrograms of folic acid) or a multivitamin that provides 100 percent of the RDA for all the B vitamins.

Clear the Cobwebs with CoQ10

Found in the mitochondria, the energy factories of our cells, coenzyme Q10 is critical for producing energy. A powerful antioxidant, CoQ10 also protects you from ever-increasing free radical attacks on mitochondria as you get older, which interfere with energy production and speed up aging.

With no known side effects, CoQ10 appears quite safe. Although you can get enough from foods, including beef, soybean oil, sardines, mackerel, and peanuts, if you still have low energy or are at risk for heart problems, you might want to supplement to see if it helps. Common medications, such as statins, antidepressants, and antihypertensives, also significantly lower levels of CoQ10. If you're on these medicines, you'll need to supplement to get enough CoQ10. Take 50 to 150 milligrams of the softgel form daily with a meal containing some fat for the best absorption.

Try Tyrosine for Mental Tiredness

Mental fatigue is linked to lower levels of L-tyrosine and other amino acids, according to a 2007 study in the *Journal of Neural Transmission*. You need tyrosine to produce the neurotransmitters dopamine, epinephrine, and norepinephrine. (Tyrosine helps make CoQ10 as well.) But stress, such as sleep deprivation and fatigue, depletes levels of these energizing substances, worsening mid- and late-life feelings of fogginess. Supplementing with tyrosine appears to increase mental focus by "reducing the acute effects of stress and fatigue on task performance," suggests a 2009 study in *Alternative Medicine Review*.

THE ANTI-FATIGUE HERB

Ashwagandha (*Withania somnifera*) is rich in phytochemicals that reduce inflammation and more and has been used in traditional Indian medicine for over 3,000 years. A 2023 study published in the *Journal of Psychopharmacology* showed that participants with stress and fatigue who took 200 milligrams of a standardized root extract of ashwagandha twice daily had significantly reduced fatigue based on the Chalder fatigue scale. A review of twelve studies in 2021 in the *Journal of Functional Morphology and Kinesiology* showed that men and women who took ashwagandha had improved performance, strength, and fitness, and reduced fatigue after exercise. Research shows it's safe to use in the short term, but if you have a medical condition, talk to your health care practitioner first before supplementing with this herb.

Other research indicates taking tyrosine can make demanding work seem easier and improve some measures of mental performance. It works quickly to boost energy and alertness (and may even brighten your mood), but tyrosine seems to work best to reinvigorate you during stressful situations.

Take tyrosine on an empty stomach. Experts recommend 500 to 1,000 milligrams daily, and although it appears safe to take indefinitely, you might want to take a monthly break to see if you can do without it. It can cause anxiety and raise blood pressure in some people, and those with melanoma or phenylketonuria should not take tyrosine.

HABIT #5
Reenergize by Finding Renewed Purpose

Once you reach mid or late life, it's best to conserve energy rather than trying to find purpose.

FALSE

Learning, challenge, and motivation are all closely linked and can hugely influence whether you feel energized or bored and fatigued. They also help keep you sharp as you get older by forming new neurons and improving brain cell communication. And whether you start with a small goal or are looking to redefine the second half of your life, pushing yourself to aim higher can fill your days with meaning and revitalize you.

Set a Goal and Feel Young Again

Motivation is one of the major components of mental energy. The motivation you get from setting and reaching a goal (so satisfying!) can invigorate you long after you've accomplished your objective, but the trick is finding one that will energize you and not seem like one more thing to cross off your to-do list. To get inspired, choose a goal that's related to something you already enjoy. Planning for and anticipating your target may help you look forward to your favorite activities even more.

For example, if you love to travel, join RoadScholar.org, a nonprofit that offers experiential all-inclusive group and solo trips with expert guides all around the world for the 50-plus crowd, and plan a trip. If you enjoy making things with your hands, whether it's knitted socks or furniture, plan a few special pieces to give as birthday or holiday gifts. Compulsive journalers or letter writers might join a writing group and try to get an essay published or start writing a memoir. Go all in and start a new business with a focus on something that's really meaningful to you.

Choosing goals with a social component can also help you maintain a strong network of supportive relationships, which protects you against energy-draining depression as you get older. If you can't wait for your weekly tennis game, set up a neighborhood tournament to raise money for a worthy cause. Like cooking? Start a supper club or take a class to master a new technique.

Goals = Energy!

Regardless of the goal you choose, expecting that you'll succeed can give you the energy you need to see it through, according to a 2009 study in the journal *Personality and Social Psychology Bulletin*. Setting high expectations can add extra motivation, and "hope can be a very powerful tool," notes Jason F. Mathers, Ph.D., a licensed psychologist in private practice. After your success, you might even be inspired to attempt a bigger challenge next time!

Break Out of a Rut to Reignite Your Zest for Life

Trying something new helps to boost energy levels. Seeing even the mundane parts of life as opportunities for fun or reward—a characteristic of the young at heart—can keep them from dragging you down and reenergize you. Try these tips to shake things up and feel years younger:

Vary Your Age-Old Routine. Even small changes such as ordering a different drink at the coffee shop or taking a different route to work once or twice a week can help you break out of a life set on automatic pilot. Novelty boosts the "feel-good" brain chemical dopamine, noted a 2006 study in the journal *Neuron.* And triggering that reward center gives you a little thrill that stimulates and energizes you and motivates you to do it again.

To counteract an energy dip during your day, switch to a new task or change your environment by going for a quick walk, even if it's just to the kitchen or a coworker's cubicle to chat for a minute. Getting up from your chair has another advantage: Movement can get your blood flowing and increase energy all by itself.

Banish boredom to changing the way you do things. For example, do your most dreaded chores while talking on the phone to your best friend. If you have a competitive nature, make a game out of work tasks or turn them into a contest with a coworker. Create an upbeat playlist or download a new podcast to listen to on your commute. Treat yourself to a favorite magazine or a back rub while waiting at the airport.

Use Perspective to Find Your Calling

All of the changes that come in mid-to-late life, such as an empty nest, retirement, taking care of aging parents, chronic illness, or feeling burned out, can make you feel adrift and listless. Adding purpose to your life can help you navigate these changes with energy to spare. J. Robert Clinton, Ph.D., a professor and author of several books about mentoring and leadership, argues that most people don't fully understand their calling—or see how their life fits into that calling—until they reach a stage he calls "convergence," which happens for many people around their fifties.

It's not easy to get to convergence, he warns, but if you're willing to reach for it, all your past challenges and successes can come together to make this stage of life incredibly rewarding and invigorating. To help you find purpose, ask yourself what your gifts, values, and passions are. Whom do you admire? How does this season fit into your larger life story? If you had unlimited time and money, what would you do to benefit others? Mulling over these questions can help clarify your calling and reenergize you to follow your heart.

Finding opportunities that line up with your core dreams and values can help you bound out of bed in the morning, eager to face the day. Experts agree that meaningful activities require both effort and using or developing your skills and talents. While work can give you a powerful sense of purpose, volunteering at something near to your heart or pursuing another passion can also bring fulfillment.

Think creatively about how you might translate your interests into purpose-filled opportunities. For example, if you get fired up about gardening, offer to start a community garden in your neighborhood or at a local school, or teach a gardening class at a community center. Ask your friends and loved ones for their suggestions as well— the outside perspective can be helpful and encouraging.

FIND PURPOSE AT MODERN ELDER ACADEMY WISDOM

Check out MEAwisdom.com, which calls itself the world's first midlife wisdom school. You'll find workshops and seminars online and in places like Baja, Mexico and Sante Fe, New Mexico to help you navigate transitions, cultivate purpose, and inspire you to make the second act of your life meaningful.

Powerful Habits: Important Dos and Don'ts to Slow the Aging Process

09

Congrats! You've learned all about the many ways that you can create positive habits for a healthy, fulfilling, long life. Here you'll find the most important do's and don'ts for longevity.

Test your Fountain of Youth IQ here >

TRUE

FALSE

(T) (F) **If you don't stop smoking in your thirties, it doesn't matter if you quit later in life.**

(T) (F) **Being sedentary can be more harmful than being overweight.**

(T) (F) **If you want to live longer—and be in good health—it's important to maintain a healthy weight.**

(T) (F) **Stress impacts your body as it's happening—it triggers fight-or-flight and a cortisol surge—but it does not cause long-term damage.**

(T) (F) **Your goal should be not just to live longer, but to live a long and healthy life free of illness and chronic disease for as long as you can.**

(T) (F) **Having a strong social network as you age makes you healthier and happier.**

HABIT #1
Don't Smoke or Vape to Live Longer and Better

If you don't stop smoking in your thirties, it doesn't matter if you quit later in life.
FALSE

It's never too late to quit and add healthy years to your life. Smokers who stop lighting up between ages thirty-five and thirty-nine live an average of six to nine years longer than they would if they continued, and quitting between ages sixty-five and sixty-nine can increase your life expectancy by one to four years, according to the American Heart Association.

Why Smoking Is So Harmful

Smoking is one of the biggest health threats we face today—not only does it shorten your life, but it can also steal quality of life in your later years. Secondhand smoke can cause respiratory infections and chronic respiratory conditions such as asthma, cancer, heart disease, and sleep disorders, and even thirdhand smoke—toxic residues, including nicotine, that linger on fabric and other surfaces—are a problem for adults and especially children.

The Centers for Disease Control and Prevention (CDC) concludes that quitting smoking and using tobacco products is the number one way to keep yourself alive (and well) longer. In the United States, one in five Americans use tobacco. There is no safe amount of smoking. If you need help quitting, talk to your doctor about resources and medications that can make it easier. Many workplaces and insurance companies also offer incentives. If you're not a smoker but are concerned about secondhand and thirdhand smoke where you work or live, contact your state representative to voice your concern or join an advocacy group (ask the tobacco coordinator at your county health department about effective local groups).

Quit Puffing to Keep Your Heart Young

Smoking ages your heart by increasing your cholesterol, raising your blood pressure, and speeding up atherosclerosis—when artery linings thicken and fatty substances and plaque block blood flow.

This increases your risk of heart attack, stroke, and other blood vessel problems. But the damage can be undone—just twenty-four hours after quitting, your blood pressure and risk of heart attack decreases. Within one year, you'll cut your risk of heart disease in half, and after fifteen years, your risk will be as low as someone who has never smoked.

THE PROBLEM WITH VAPING

Often smokers turn to vaping, thinking that's probably safer. E-cigarettes—which work by heating nicotine and other compounds so that you can inhale them—do contain fewer chemicals. A regular cigarette contains over 7,000 of them, many of which are toxic. But in 2020, according to the CDC, there were over 2,807 cases of lung injury attributed to e-cigarette or vaping use-associated lung injury (EVALI) and sixty-eight deaths. This may be due to the vitamin E acetate in e-cigarette vaping pods or cartridges. Research at Johns Hopkins University published in *Chemical Research in Toxicology* in 2021 showed that there are industrial chemicals in e-cigs that could have adverse effects. Data links e-cigarettes to lung disease, asthma, and cardiovascular disease. Rather than using e-cigarettes to wean yourself off of traditional ones, it's better to use smoking cessation products.

Long Live Your Lungs!

Your lungs have a natural defense system to protect them, but cigarette smoke interferes with that protection and leaves you vulnerable to infection and disease. Tobacco smoke can narrow your airways, making breathing more difficult, and cause chronic inflammation and swelling, eventually destroying lung cells and setting off changes that can grow into cancer. In a group of similarly aged volunteers, smokers' lungs appeared an average of ten years older than nonsmokers' (and five years older than past smokers'), according to a 2009 study by Japanese researchers.

Smoking leads to breathing problems such as asthma, bronchitis, emphysema, and chronic obstructive pulmonary disease (COPD). And it's directly responsible for about 90 percent of deaths due to lung cancer, according to the American Lung Association. Ten years after quitting, however, your risk of dying from lung cancer is almost the same as someone who has never smoked. Quitting can also immediately improve your breathing and other smoking-related lung problems, including COPD.

Save Your Skin from Premature Aging

Not only does the repetitive motion of pursing your lips around a cigarette cause wrinkles around your mouth, but a 2007 study in the *Archives of Dermatology* found that smoking causes skin to age faster. The study's authors also noted that the more packs people smoked per day, the older-looking their skin was.

Smoking breaks down collagen and inhibits your skin from making more, leading to inelasticity and wrinkling. It also causes blood vessels to shrink so your skin doesn't get as much oxygen; over time that hurts skin's ability to heal and leaves you with a not-so-lovely yellowish tone. Quit lighting up for good, however, and you can reduce these signs of aging, even if you've smoked for years. Secondhand smoke has similar effects, so avoid it as much as possible, too.

> **KEEP YOUR TEETH AND GUMS HEALTHY FOR LIFE**
>
> Smoking may be responsible for nearly 75 percent of periodontal diseases among adults, notes the American Dental Association. But ten years after quitting, your risk of gum disease is the same as that of nonsmokers.
>
> ___ Poor oral health, and particularly gum disease, can age your whole body. However, keeping your gums and teeth in tip-top shape can potentially protect you from heart disease, stroke, diabetes, cancer, and even cognitive decline as you get older. Researchers aren't sure why or how oral health affects the rest of your body, but early evidence indicates the bacteria that cause gum disease also cause chronic inflammation. In addition, the bacteria buildup (or plaque) can enter the bloodstream and release toxins throughout the body.
>
> ___ A 2008 New York University study showed that daily brushing and flossing reduced the amount of gum disease–causing bacteria in the mouth after just two weeks. The American Dental Association (ADA) recommends brushing at least twice a day for two minutes at a time. Replace your toothbrush every three to four months, or sooner if the bristles start fraying.
>
> ___ An 11-year study published in 2019 in the *Journal of Clinical Periodontology* showed clear benefits from using an electric toothbrush, including less tooth decay and healthier gums. Study participants also kept their teeth longer. You should also floss at least once daily (if you have gum disease, your dentist may recommend flossing more frequently). Limit sweets and avoid all forms of tobacco too.

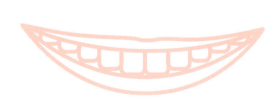

HABIT #2
Conquer Couch Potato Syndrome to Stay Fit for Life

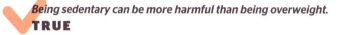

Being sedentary can be more harmful than being overweight.
TRUE

Research shows that, in terms of maintaining health and staying young, being sedentary can be more harmful than being overweight, although they're often linked. But inactivity affects far more than your waistline. Prolonged sitting is also strongly associated with a decreased ability to process blood sugar, diabetes, metabolic syndrome, cardiovascular disease, and cancer, as well as overall risk of death, point out the authors of a 2010 editorial in the *British Journal of Sports Medicine*.

Being sedentary for long stretches during the day puts you at risk for all those problems even if you work out several times a week. In fact, the study authors suggest redefining sedentary to mean periods of muscular inactivity rather than the absence of exercise, so that people don't think they can go for a thirty-minute walk and then stay stationary the rest of the day. Both everyday movement and regular exercise are critical to keeping you young and healthy.

Increase Your Everyday Activity Levels to Stay Youthful

Yes, as you age, you can become less active than when you were younger. But you can fight that natural tendency to slow down by intentionally finding ways to move more. Here's how:

Small movements count. Standing and stretching, going up the stairs to grab a coffee, or delivering a memo in person to break up long periods of sitting is helpful.

If you find yourself glued to your computer, set an alarm to go off every forty-five minutes or so to remind you to get up and stretch your legs.

Stuck in a car? You can safely stretch your arms and periodically contract and release your leg muscles or rotate your ankles to keep your blood flowing.

If TV ties you to the couch, be warned: The more TV you watch, the higher your waist circumference, blood pressure, and other markers of heart and metabolic diseases (such as diabetes) are likely to be.

> **MAKE IT A HABIT: GET OFF THE COUCH**
>
> Limit your tube time to shows you really care about, and exercise while you watch. If you work at a computer, get up and walk around for a few minutes once an hour. Try interval training, with bursts of speed separated by moments of rest.

Exercise Smarter for Longer Life

Exercise can give you longer telomeres, the small pieces of DNA that protect the ends of your chromosomes and shrink with age. Scientists consider their length a good indicator of aging (regardless of how old the calendar says you are). A sedentary lifestyle is linked to shorter telomeres in white blood cells and may accelerate the aging process, reports a 2008 study in the *Archives of Internal Medicine*. However, other studies show that exercise regulates the proteins that stabilize telomeres and keep them from degrading, while protecting against stress-related cell death. Aerobic exercise and strength training can also increase endurance, muscle strength, and balance, making it easier to be active in other areas of your life. Research confirms that regular exercisers also move more in their leisure time.

Get Your Exercise In

Experts recommend doing at least thirty minutes of moderate-intensity exercise on most or all days of the week. An even more effective approach might be interval training, or alternating periods of high effort with rest, which allows you to reap the benefits of exercise in less time. A 2008 study in *Applied Physiology, Nutrition, and Metabolism* found that high-intensity interval training (ten four-minute sprints separated by two minutes of rest) three days a week for six weeks improved fat burning, endurance, oxygen use, and strength. Research suggests it can also increase speed. Intense bursts of activity appear to enhance aerobic capacity, boost blood vessel function, build muscle, lower blood sugar, and improve insulin response more effectively than a workout of continuous moderate exercise. Because they're so challenging, intervals can also rev up a sluggish midlife metabolism longer post-workout than steady, lower-intensity exercise. Interval training can be strenuous, so ask your doctor if it's safe for you before trying it.

HABIT #3
Don't Let Your BMI Creep Too High in Midlife

If you want to live longer—and be in good health—it's important to maintain a healthy weight.
TRUE

Overwhelming evidence indicates that if you want to live longer—and be in good health—keeping your weight in check is one of the most important steps you can take. When you're overweight, nearly every system in your body has to work harder to keep functioning, and the extra pounds throw your neuroendocrine system off balance. Fat cells produce hormones that raise your risk of type 2 diabetes, along with inflammatory substances that stiffen your arteries, heart, and other organs. In addition, excess weight can actually change your heart and blood vessel structure and function, and to meet increased metabolic needs, circulating blood volume, plasma volume, and cardiac output all increase. Thanks to those effects (and others), obesity ultimately increases your risk of stroke, cancer, heart disease, high blood pressure, sleep disorders, and type 2 diabetes over time.

> **HOW TO CALCULATE YOUR BMI**
>
> Researchers frequently use BMI to investigate how weight affects health. You can find a BMI calculator online, or you can measure it yourself by dividing your weight in kilograms by the square of your height in meters (kg/m^2).
>
> Overweight is defined as having a BMI between 25 and 30, while a BMI of 30 or higher translates to obesity (or being about 30 pounds [14 kg] overweight for a 5'4" [1.62 m] woman).

Avoid Diabetes

Diabetes speeds up aging throughout your body and increases your risk of other unwelcome health problems, lowering your quality of life as you get older. Remarkably, diabetes diagnoses have doubled over the past thirty years, mostly in people with a BMI over 30.

In fact, the Nurses' Health Study found that obesity was the most powerful predictor of diabetes—women with a BMI over 35 were nearly thirty-nine times more likely to develop diabetes than women with a BMI of less than 23, according to a 2010 report in the journal *Circulation*. All told, the researchers note, forty-year-olds who weigh too much shorten their life expectancy by more than three years.

Stay Slim as You Get Older

Maintaining a stable, healthy weight throughout midlife may benefit you even more than whether you're lean as an older adult. Researchers following more than 17,000 women for several decades found that those who gained the least amount of weight over the course of the study were not only more likely to live to age seventy, but also to be free of eleven major chronic illnesses (including heart disease, cancer, stroke, and Parkinson's disease) and have no substantial cognitive, physical, or mental limitations.

And while being obese at age fifty increased their risk for health problems by 79 percent, what happened to the women's weight between ages eighteen and fifty mattered most, according to the 2009 study in the *British Medical Journal.* Those who had a BMI over 25 (considered overweight) at age eighteen and gained 22 pounds (10 kg) or more had the lowest odds of reaching seventy in good health. So if you're under fifty and you've noticed the number on the scale creeping up year after year, put a stop to it now to improve your chances of living a long, healthy life. Of course, it's never too late to improve your well-being by slimming down if you're overweight.

Lose Weight to Live Longer

Lean people (with a BMI less than 25) cut their risk of premature death in half compared to those who are obese (a BMI over 30), according to a 2004 study in the *New England Journal of Medicine.* Accordingly, experts recommend keeping your BMI between 19 and 24. See the tips in chapter 2 to help you slim down or maintain a healthy weight as you get older, or ask your doctor for suggestions.

AVOID THE STANDARD AMERICAN DIET TO KEEP YOUR BODY YOUNG

Americans are big on snacks, sweets, and processed convenience foods, but as you get older and your metabolism slows, you need fewer calories to maintain your weight. That means there's less room in your diet for non-nutritious foods like these.

——**Excess sodium** causes your body to retain fluid, leading to hypertension and making your heart work harder. Experts recommend limiting your daily sodium intake to 2,300 milligrams (1 teaspoon [6 g] of table salt), but you'll likely find that eating processed or prepared foods takes you past that limit in no time.

——**Saturated and trans fats** increase inflammation that ages your brain, heart, immune system, and even your skin. You need some saturated fat, found in animal products such as meat and full-fat dairy, but experts advise keeping your intake to less than 7 percent of your daily calories. Shun products with trans fats—shortening or partially hydrogenated oils—as much as possible.

——**Added sugars**, such as high-fructose corn syrup, are found in an astonishing array of packaged foods. They provide empty calories and send your blood sugar levels soaring, stimulating the production of advanced glycation end products (AGEs), which increase free radicals and inflammation. Continually spiking your blood sugar with sweets also triggers the release of extra insulin, which research shows turns off a "longevity gene" in your body.

——Following the Mediterranean diet and cooking meals at home is a great way to avoid "junk" foods and get the nutrition you need for health and longevity.

> **MAKE IT A HABIT:**
> **LOSE EXCESS WEIGHT AND KEEP IT OFF**
>
> Shedding even a few pounds can help restore a youthful figure, trim your medical bills, and add healthy years to your life. Losing as little as 5 percent of your body weight can reduce your risk of chronic illness. Avoiding junk foods and cooking Mediterranean diet meals improve health and longevity.

HABIT #4
Steer Clear of Chronic Stress to Prevent Premature Aging

Stress impacts your body as it's happening—it triggers fight-or-flight and a cortisol surge—but it does not cause long-term damage.

FALSE

Chronic stress actually changes your brain structure, which may make it harder for your brain to "turn off" the stress response over time. That's worrisome because too much tension speeds up aging by increasing free radical attacks, exposing your body to a continual flood of stress hormones such as cortisol, degrading your thymus gland and weakening your immune system, reducing cell communication, and creating constant low-grade inflammation. Chronic stress also leads to premature aging of key body systems that help you adapt to stress and respond to stressful challenges.

Continually high levels of cortisol can reduce bone density and trigger shifts in body composition as well, reducing muscle and encouraging fat to settle around your middle. That can put you at risk for osteoporosis, metabolic syndrome, and diabetes. Stress also accelerates some biomarkers of aging, including shrinking your telomeres, the protective caps on the ends of chromosomes. Telomeres naturally shorten every time a cell divides, and when they get short enough the cell dies, which may cause or contribute to some age-related diseases.

In addition to physical wear and tear, anxiety can also take a toll on your mental and emotional health. For instance, stress may make older adults more prone to depression, which is linked to cognitive decline, and it can also drain your energy and keep you from appreciating life's pleasures. However, research suggests that lifestyle changes such as exercise, diet, and social support can actually reverse the brain changes brought on by chronic stress. That means managing stress can lengthen your life span while increasing your quality of life, allowing you to enjoy the healthy years to come.

Exercise to Tame Tension as You Age

It bears repeating that exercise is one of the best ways to beat stress. It can help you burn off extra physical and mental energy, boost feel-good neurotransmitters to lift your mood, and help you sleep better. It also directly counteracts some of the harmful effects of chronic stress that age you beyond your years, including strengthening your muscles and bones, keeping you trim, recharging your immune system, and warding off depression.

In addition, exercise can actually slow the shrinking of your telomeres and protect them against stress-related cell death, according to a 2009 study in the journal *Circulation*. It also helps your body adapt to stress and be more resilient over time.

Interestingly, the stress response activates the reward center of the brain, along with the adrenals, the nervous system, and the pain relief areas. The reward is the relief you experience once the stress has passed. One reason why physical activity works so well to alleviate anxiety is because many people report the same thing with exercise—they may not enjoy doing it, but they feel so much better afterward that the promise of reward is enough to get them to lace up their sneakers.

> **MAKE IT A HABIT: MANAGE CHRONIC STRESS WELL**
>
> Make sure you sleep well, eat a good diet, and get regular exercise. Don't worry; change your perceptions of stressors by practicing acceptance and taking one day at a time. Pursue social connections and spirituality to help buffer the harmful effects of stress. If stress is interfering with your daily routine, activities, or relationships, consider seeing a therapist who is trained in cognitive behavioral therapy (CBT) or acceptance and commitment therapy (ACT) to help you to change the way you react to stress.

Change Your Perception of Stress to Slow Aging

You may not be able to eliminate chronic stressors, such as financial stress or caregiving, but you can change how you react to them. In addition to regular exercise and a healthy diet, sleep and good coping strategies are also critical. Restorative sleep can help refresh your perspective and make stressors seem easier to deal with. And healthy older adults practice acceptance, not worrying, and taking things one day at a time to cope with their stress, notes a 2001 study in the *Journal of Aging and Health*. Research also shows that maintaining strong social ties, pursuing religious and spiritual beliefs, managing your expectations and goals, and participating in activities you find meaningful can reduce stress and its harmful effects.

Practice the Relaxation Response

Additionally, you can teach yourself to elicit the relaxation response instead of staying constantly on edge. Try meditation, breathing exercises, yoga, biofeedback training, or even stroking a beloved pet. While doing these activities in the face of a stressor can help you calm down in the moment, practicing them regularly can retrain your parasympathetic nervous system, which helps you feel more relaxed, to be in charge more of the time.

Be in the moment. Grounding yourself in the now helps reduce stress because you're in the present moment without the burden of the past and future. Try to focus on one item from your to-do list at a time, rather than piling on everything all at once, can reduce overwhelm. Whatever you're doing, whether it's working on a project, helping your kids, or having lunch with a friend, try to just be there rather than thinking about what you need to do next. For more help check out *The Power of Now* by Eckhart Tolle.

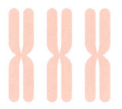

HABIT #5
Don't Let Your Genes Shorten Your Life

Your goal should be not just to live longer, but to live a long and healthy life free of illness and chronic disease for as long as you can.
TRUE

When you think about antiaging, your goal shouldn't be just to live a long life. You also want to embrace a concept called *compression of morbidity,* or delaying the onset of age-related illnesses and chronic conditions until very late in life to ensure you can enjoy and be active in your later years. If you have a family history of heart disease, cancer, diabetes, Alzheimer's, or other conditions, your risk of getting those diseases increases. Likewise, if you have a close relative who lived healthfully to old age, your odds of doing the same go up. However, your genes don't tell the whole story. Certain lifestyle factors, such as diet and exercise, can change how you express those genes, influencing whether you develop certain diseases and how severe they are as you get older.

Minimize "Inflamm-aging"

As you get older, natural levels of inflammatory substances increase, leaving you with chronic low-grade inflammation that scientists have dubbed "inflamm-aging." A 2006 study in the *Annals of the New York Academy of Sciences* noted that chronic inflammation promotes or exacerbates age-related conditions such as cardiovascular diseases, atherosclerosis, Alzheimer's disease, arthritis, muscle loss, and type 2 diabetes, among others. The researchers found that the increased inflammation by itself is not enough to trigger those diseases and to shorten life. However, if you have a genetic predisposition to specific age-related diseases and also to strong inflammatory responses, chronic low-grade inflammation can cause real problems.

To keep inflamm-aging under control, eat an anti-inflammatory diet and maintain a healthy weight as you get older. Body fat is hormonally active tissue, and it is one of the main sources of the inflammatory substances such as C-reactive protein and interleukin-6 that play a role in age-accelerating diseases such as atherosclerosis, insulin resistance, and diabetes.

Reduce Insulin Resistance to Halt Premature Aging

Insulin controls the processing, storage, and distribution of energy, and disruptions in its production or response can lead to obesity and diabetes, aging of body tissues, and possibly even cancer. Insulin resistance, or problems with insulin response and blood sugar metabolism, promotes oxidative stress and inflammation, both linked to premature aging, according to a 2010 study by Italian researchers.

Animal studies suggest that altering genes involved in the insulin/insulin-like growth factor (IGF-1) signaling pathway can extend animal life span. IGF-1 regulates cell growth and development, especially in nerve cells, and high levels are linked to cancer. In humans, studies that have looked at centenarians found that they generally have preserved insulin responsiveness and low levels of IGF-1 in their blood. Insulin resistance is more common as you get older, thanks in part to shifts in body composition to less muscle and more fat. But you can keep insulin functioning properly and slow aging by avoiding swings in blood sugar and building muscle through exercise—particularly strength training. Exercise also uses glucose for energy so less can build up in your system, and it helps your cells become more sensitive to insulin.

Fight Free Radicals to Live Longer

Genes that counteract oxidative stress, such as superoxide dismutase and paraoxonase (PON1), may also help you live longer. PON1 activity decreases significantly during aging, while free radical attacks generally multiply. Unstable free radicals steal electrons from nearby molecules, ravaging them and speeding up aging. Chronic oxidative stress contributes to age-related changes in immune function and other regulatory systems, such as the nervous and endocrine systems, as well as the

> **MAKE IT A HABIT: GO BEYOND GENETICS**
>
> Calm inflammation by maintaining a healthy weight and eating an anti-inflammatory diet. Avoid spikes in blood sugar and exercise regularly to prevent insulin resistance. Fight aging free radicals by consuming plenty of antioxidant-rich foods.

LOOKING FOR THE FOUNTAIN OF YOUTH

In 2024, researchers at the Albert Einstein College of Medicine who've scanned the genomes of centenarians (less than 1 percent of people live this long or older) to find the genes that enable long life found fifteen longevity variants. The five-year study focused on 450 participants ninety-five and older who are enrolled in Einstein's Longevity Genes Product and compared them to the genomes of 550 people aged 70 with no family history of extreme longevity. The research will continue through 2029, thanks to a grant from NIH. The goal is to identify these longevity variants and use them to develop drugs that mimic their effects to prevent age-related diseases so that people can live longer, healthier lives.

communication between them, according to a 2009 study in *Current Pharmaceutical Design*. To decrease oxidative stress and lengthen your life span, the study's authors suggest getting an abundance of antioxidants through diet. Brightly colored fruits and vegetables (aim for five to nine servings per day), red wine, green and black tea, dark chocolate, and beans are all good sources.

HABIT #6
Build and Maintain a Strong Social Network to Live Longer

Having a strong social network as you age makes you healthier and happier.
TRUE

People with a strong social network live an average of 22 percent longer than those without one, according to a 2005 study in the *Journal of Epidemiology and Community Health* that followed nearly 1,500 people for ten years. Why are social ties so beneficial? For one thing, having close friendships protects against depression, which is increasingly common as you get older. That, in turn, may motivate you to take better care of yourself.

Having a network of people you can turn to in times of stress or anxiety can also give you support and practical help, ultimately minimizing stress. Plus, loved ones watch your back and push you to see a doctor if you need to. Social connection keeps you physically active as well. A 2009 study in the *Archives of Internal Medicine* found that older adults who were less social had a more rapid decline in motor function. The adults measured their social activeness on a scale of one to five, with one meaning they participated in social activities once a year, and five indicating near-daily participation. For every one-point drop in their scores, their physical function declined 33 percent—equivalent to being five years older than their actual age. If their scores dropped by a point in a single year, the resulting physical decline led to a 65 percent increased risk of disability and 40 percent increased chance of dying.

Note that studies show health benefits for a *strong* social network—not necessarily a *large* one. While having a diverse group of acquaintances, casual friends, close friends, and those who are like family (they might even be family) is beneficial, research suggests that those top two tiers are most important to your well-being.

For example, while younger people may have larger overall social circles, both young and older adults tend to have the same number of close connections, which they agree is what helps them feel socially engaged. In fact, as relationships in the outer social circle dwindle, older adults may find themselves able to devote more time to close emotional ties and focus on those meaningful relationships. Having fewer than three very close relationships, however, is associated with loneliness, anxiety, and depression. If you've dipped below that, consider investing in other relationships to find another true friend or two.

BANISH THE ENERGY VAMPIRES FROM YOUR LIFE

It's healthy to surround yourself with people who make you feel good, but some relationships drain your life force and can detract from the good ones that will keep you healthy, happy, and energized as you get older. It can be hard to let go, so first take a clear-eyed look at your history together to determine if you can salvage the bond by setting (and keeping!) limits, or if you're better off ending the relationship. If you can't—like with family or coworkers—learn coping skills like setting wise boundaries.

> **MAKE IT A HABIT: STRENGTHEN YOUR SOCIAL CONNECTIONS**
>
> Regularly interact with friends and loved ones to live a long, healthy, and happy life. Have at least three close relationships with friends or family members to protect against loneliness, anxiety, and depression. Nurture existing relationships while developing new ones.

Put Yourself Out There for the Long Haul

If your social circle is shrinking, you may need to make an extra effort to meet new people and stay engaged. Whether it's taking a class, volunteering, joining a jogging group, or attending a lecture at your local community center, there are countless opportunities to get involved and make new friends. Cast a wide social net, and be open to new places, people, and experiences. These things can be helpful for deepening existing relationships as well, and the combination of social activity and novelty can also help ward off cognitive decline and boost fading energy levels as you get older.

Pursue Faith for a More Meaningful Life

Being part of a faith community might also add years to your life—several studies have found that religious participation is linked to longevity. A 1999 study in the journal *Demography* found that white people who attended religious services at least once a week lived seven years longer than those who never attended—and black people lived an impressive fourteen years longer.

The benefit partly stems from social connection and having a place to engage in leisure activities that are cognitively stimulating and encourage physical activity, notes a 2008 study in the *Journals of Gerontology: Psychological Sciences and Social Sciences*. Early research also suggests that religious men and women, regardless of race or ethnicity, tend to engage in healthier lifestyles. And a 2000 study in the *International Journal of Psychiatry in Medicine* found that for women, attending religious services once a week protected their health just as much as avoiding cigarette smoking, doing regular physical activity, limiting alcohol consumption, and participating in nonreligious social involvement.

It doesn't have to be a religious service; spiritual and meditation centers, Unity churches, and other nondenominational organizations promote faith, mindfulness, positive thinking, and more, and can also provide socialization, support, and connection.

INDEX

A

acupuncture, *74, 75*
aerobic exercise, *36, 97, 118*
aging
  antioxidants and, *154, 155*
  energy vampires, *156*
  faith and, *157*
  genetics and, *153-155*
  Longevity Genes Product, *155*
  mental health and, *151-153*
  sedentary living, *147-148*
  smoking, *144-146*
  social connections and, *155-157*
  stress, *151-153*
  vaping, *144-146*
  weight management, *148-151*
alcohol
  blood pressure and, *81*
  bones and joints and, *69*
  brain health and, *51*
American diet, *150*
anger management, *84, 86*
antioxidants
  aging and, *154, 155*
  brain health and, *44, 45, 46, 56-57*
  energy and, *134, 135, 138*
  heart health and, *81-82, 88, 89*
  immune system and, *102, 103, 104, 105*
  skin and, *17, 18, 23*
ArginMax, *126*
aromatherapy, *93, 94, 117, 137*
ashwagandha, *136, 138*
astragalus, *106-107*

B

balance, *39, 41*
biotin, *26*
blood pressure
  alcohol and, *81*
  exercise and, *79, 81*
  nutrition and, *79, 80*
  sexual health and, *111, 112*
  sodium and, *80*
blood sugar. *See diabetes*
BMI calculation, *149*
bones and joints
  acupuncture and, *74, 75*
  alcohol and, *69*
  Boswellia extract, *73*
  fruits and, *64*
  massage therapy, *75*
  muscle and, *60*
  natural remedies and, *70*
  nutrition and, *61, 63-67, 68*
  pain, *70, 71-72, 74, 75*
  processed foods and, *68*
  Pycnogenol, *72-73*
  S-adenosylmethionine (SAM-e), *71-72*

  sexual health and, *110*
  sugar and, *68, 69*
  transcutaneous electrical nerve stimulation (TENS), *74*
  vegetables and, *64*
  weight and, *60-62*
Boswellia extract, *73*
Botox, *27*
brain health. *See also mental health*
  antioxidants, *44, 45, 46, 56-57*
  CoQ10, *57*
  cognition, *54-55*
  depression, *47-49*
  exercise and, *48, 49*
  focus, *52-53*
  forest bathing, *50*
  ginkgo biloba, *57*
  mind-body relaxation, *53*
  nutrition and, *44-47, 56-57*
  puzzles, *55*
  routine and, *54, 55*
  sleep and, *51*
  stress and, *49-50*
  supplements for, *56, 57*
  vitamin B12 and, *56*
  wine and, *46*

C

caffeine, *30-31, 69, 135*
calcium, *63, 64, 65, 67, 68*
capsaicin, *30*
chemical peels, *24*
cholesterol
  exercise and, *79*
  fiber and, *83*
  nutrition and, *78-80, 83*
  statins, *88, 111*
chondroitin, *70-71*
coenzyme Q10 (CoQ10), *57, 88, 89, 138*
cognition, *54-55*
collagen, *12, 13, 14, 18, 19, 21, 22, 23, 25, 27*
compression of morbidity, *153*
convergence, *141*
cortisol, *22, 32*
curcumin, *45-46*

D

depression. *See also mental health*
  exercise and, *48, 49*
  sleep and, *51*
  social connections and, *86*
  social support for, *49*
  volunteering and, *86*
dermatologists, *27*

diabetes
  insulin resistance, *154*
  medications for, *88*
  sexual health and, *110, 112*
  sugar intake and, *83*
  weight and, *149*
  whole grains and, *47*

E

echinacea, *107*
elderberry, *107*
endorphins, *33*
energy
  antioxidants, *134, 135, 138*
  aromatherapy, *137*
  ashwagandha, *136, 138*
  cold water and, *132*
  convergence, *141*
  CoQ10, *138*
  energy vampires, *156*
  exercise and, *133*
  extra activities, *133*
  fatigue, *132*
  mental health and, *130-131*
  mental vs. physical fatigue, *132*
  multitasking, *130, 131*
  Newton's law and, *132*
  nutrition and, *134-135*
  purpose and, *139-141*
  routine and, *140*
  sexual health and, *121*
  stress and, *130-131*
  supplements for, *136-139*
  tea vs. coffee, *135*
  tyrosine, *138-139*
  vitamin B, *136-137*
epigallocatechin gallate (EGCG), *30*
exercise
  balance and, *39, 41*
  blood pressure and, *79, 81*
  cholesterol and, *79*
  depression and, *48, 49*
  energy and, *133*
  fatigue and, *133*
  as habit, *36*
  immune system and, *97*
  intensity of, *36, 38*
  Kegels, *119*
  mood and, *21*
  nonexercise activity thermogenesis (NEAT), *38*
  random opportunities for, *133*
  sedentary living, *147-148*
  sexual health and, *114, 118-119*
  skin and, *22*
  strength training, *37, 119*
  stress and, *21, 22*
  tracker, *40*
  variety of, *41*

F

face yoga, *21*
facial massage, *23*
faith, *157*
fermented foods, *62, 66, 67*
fiber, *83, 134*
focus, *52–53*
food. *See nutrition*
forest bathing, *50*
free radicals, *154–155*

G

galangal, *46*
genetics, *153–155*
ghrelin, *34*
ginger, *30, 46*
gingerols, *30*
ginkgo, *57, 126*
ginseng, *105–106, 127*
glucosamine, *70–71*
glycosaminoglycans, *70*
gratitude, *100–101*
green tea, *30–31*
grudges, *99*

H

hair, *25–26*
heart health
anger management, *84, 86*
antioxidants, *81–82, 88, 89*
cholesterol and, *78–80*
CoQ10, *88, 89*
fiber and, *83*
mental health and, *84–87*
nutrition and, *79, 81–83*
omega-3 fatty acids, *87, 89*
statins, *88*
stress management, *86–87*
vitamin B and, *82*
high-intensity focused ultra
sound facial (HIFU), *27*
humidity, *15*
hyaluronic acid, *13*

I

immune system
aerobic exercise and, *97*
antioxidants, *102, 103, 104, 105*
astragalus, *106–107*
echinacea, *107*
elderberry, *107*
ginseng, *105–106*
laughter and, *93*
massage and, *94*
mental health and, *98–101*
music and, *93*
nutrition and, *102–104*
positivity and, *98–101*
probiotics, *104*
selenium, *104*
sleep and, *95–97*
supplements for, *105–107*
support practices, *92–93*
thymus gland, *92*
touch and, *94*

yoga and, *93*
zinc, *104*
inflammation
bones and joints and, *68–69*
brain health and, *44–47*
immune system and, *92, 93,
94, 95*
"inflamm-aging," *153–154*
natural remedies for, *70, 72, 73*
vitamin B, *82*
weight and, *62*
insulin, *35, 83, 134, 154*

J

joints. *See bones and joints*

K

Kegels, *119*

L

laser skin treatments, *27*
laughter, *87, 93, 100, 131*
leptin, *34*
lip gloss, *25*
lipids, *13, 15, 16, 26*

M

maca root, *127*
magnesium, *65, 67*
massage
bones and joints and, *75*
facial massage, *23*
immune system and, *94*
meditation
brain health and, *52–53*
sexual health and, *116*
stress and, *33*
Yoga Nidra, *19*
Mediterranean diet, *44,
62, 134, 150*
melanocytes, *25*
mental health. *See also
brain health; depression;
stress*
energy and, *130–131*
gratitude, *100–101*
grudges, *99*
heart health and, *84–87*
immune system and, *98–101*
meditation and, *52–53*
mindfulness, *115–117, 153*
positivity, *98–101*
purpose and, *139–141*
sexual health and, *120–121*
social support, *49, 86*
metabolism, *30, 31, 38*
microdermabrasion, *23, 24*
microneedling, *23*
mind-body relaxation, *53*
Modern Elder Academy, *141*
muscle
balance and, *39, 41*
bones and joints and, *60*
metabolism and, *36*
strength training, *37*

N

nonexercise activity
thermogenesis (NEAT), *38*
nutrition
American diet, *150*
antioxidants, *103–104*
blood pressure and, *79, 80*
bones and joints and, *61,
63–67, 68*
brain health and, *44–47, 56–57*
caffeine, *30–31, 69, 135*
calcium, *63, 64, 65, 67, 68*
cholesterol and, *78–80*
curcumin, *45–46*
diabetes and, *83*
energy and, *134–135*
fermented foods, *62, 66, 67*
fish, *44, 45*
ginger, *30*
green tea, *30–31*
heart health and, *79, 81–83*
immune system and, *102–104*
magnesium, *65, 67*
Mediterranean diet, *44, 62,
134, 150*
metabolism and, *30, 31*
omega-3 fatty acids, *12, 16, 18,
44, 87, 89*
omega-6 fatty acids, *16, 18*
organic foods, *45, 46*
peppers, *30*
pesticides, *46*
phytonutrients, *44, 45*
potassium, *65*
processed foods, *68*
proteins, *31*
sexual health and, *127*
skin health and, *17, 18*
sodium, *68, 80, 150*
stress and, *32–33*
sugar, *68, 69, 83*
superfoods, *45*
tea, *135*
thermogenesis, *30*
vitamin B, *26, 56, 82, 127, 136–137*
vitamin C, *65*
vitamin D, *65, 66, 102*
vitamin K2, *65, 67*
whole grains, *47*
zinc, *18, 104*

O

omega-3 fatty acids, *12, 16,
18, 44, 87, 89*
omega-6 fatty acids, *16, 18*
organic foods, *45, 46*

P

pain
bones and joints, *70, 71–72, 74, 75*
flexibility and, *39*
sexual health and, *110*
weight and, *61, 62*
peppers, *30*
peptides, *14*
pesticides, *46*
phytonutrients, *44, 45*

polymethyl methacrylate (PMMA), 27
polyphenols, 46
potassium, 65
probiotics, 104
proteins
energy and, 134
exercise and, 148
hair and, 26
metabolism and, 31
muscle and, 31, 61
puzzles, 55
Pycnogenol, 72–73

R

red light therapy (RLT), 22–23
religion, 157
resveratrol, 46
Retin-A, 14, 24
rotation of consciousness, 19

S

S-adenosylmethionine (SAM-e), 71–72
salt, 68, 80, 150
sedentary living, 147–148
selenium, 18, 104
sexual health
aerobic exercise and, 118
aging and, 122
ArginMax, 126
blood pressure and, 111, 112
communication and, 122–125
confidence and, 112–114
diabetes and, 110
energy and, 121
exercise and, 114, 118–119
fatigue and, 121
ginkgo, 126–127
ginseng, 127
immune system and, 94
joint pain and, 110
Kegels, 119
maca root, 127
medications and, 111
mental health and, 120–121
mindfulness and, 115–117
nonsexual intimacy, 123
nutrition and, 127
pain and, 110
routine and, 121
sensory mindfulness, 117
statins and, 111
strength training and, 119
stress and, 120–121
supplements for, 126–127
testosterone, 119
vitamin B, 127
yoga and, 116
skin health
antioxidants, 17, 18, 23
Botox, 27
breathing practices and, 21
chemical peels, 24

collagen, 12, 13, 14, 18, 19, 21, 22, 23, 25, 27
exercise and, 22
face yoga, 21
facial massage, 23
fillers, 27
high-intensity focused ultrasound facial (HIFU), 27
humidity, 15
hyaluronic acid, 13
laser treatments, 27
lip gloss, 25
lipids, 13
microdermabrasion, 23, 24
microneedling, 23
nutrients and, 17, 18
omega-3 fatty acids, 12, 16, 18
omega-6 fatty acids, 16, 18
peptides, 14
polymethyl methacrylate (PMMA), 27
red light therapy (RLT), 22–23
Retin-A, 14, 24
selenium, 18
stress and, 19–20, 20
sun damage, 12, 102
sunglasses, 15
sunscreens, 12
zinc and, 18
sleep
depression and, 51
immune system and, 95–97
insulin and, 35
journaling, 96
natural remedies for, 97
strategies for, 96
tips for, 35
weight and, 34–35
smoking, 144–146
social connections
aging and, 155–157
depression and, 49, 86
sodium 68, 80, 150
sodium hyaluronate.
See hyaluronic acid
statins, 88, 111
strength training, 37
stress. *See also* mental health
brain health and, 49–50
cortisol, 32
curcumin and, 45–46
energy and, 130–131
exercise and, 21, 22
management techniques, 33, 49, 86–87
meditation and, 33
nutrition and, 32–33
skin and, 19–20, 20
weight gain and, 32
Yoga Nidra ("yogic sleep"), 19
sugar
bones and joints and, 68, 69
consumption of, 83
sun damage. *See skin health*
sunscreens, 12
superfoods, 45

supplements
brain health, 56, 57
energy supplements, 136–139
immune system and, 105–107
sexual health and, 126–127

tea, 135
teeth, 24–25, 26
testosterone, 119
thermogenesis, 30
thymus gland, 92
transcutaneous electrical nerve stimulation (TENS), 74

vaping, 144–146
vitamin B, 26, 56, 82, 127, 136–137
vitamin C, 65
vitamin D, 65, 66, 102
vitamin K2, 65, 67
volunteering, 86

weight
BMI management, 148–151
bones and joints and, 60–62
diabetes and, 149
inflammation and, 62
insulin and, 35
life expectancy and, 150
sleep and, 34–35
stress and, 32–33
weight training, 37
whole grains, 47
wine, 46

yoga
immune system and, 93
mindfulness, 116–117
sexual health and, 116
Yoga Nidra ("yogic sleep"), 19

Z

zinc, 18, 104